T AND ME

T AND ME

Journey into Discovery

Mary Burgess-Smith, Ph.D.
Co-written with Peg Campbell

iUniverse, Inc.
New York Bloomington Shanghai

T and Me

Journey into Discovery

iUniverse books may be ordered through booksellers or by contacting:

iUniverse
1663 Liberty Drive
Bloomington, IN 47403
www.iuniverse.com
1-800-Authors (1-800-288-4677)

Because of the dynamic nature of the Internet, any Web addresses or links contained in this book may have changed since publication and may no longer be valid.

The information, ideas, and suggestions in this book are not intended as a substitute for professional medical advice. Before following any suggestions contained in this book, you should consult your personal physician. Neither the author nor the publisher shall be liable or responsible for any loss or damage allegedly arising as a consequence of your use or application of any information or suggestions in this book.

ISBN: 978-0-595-48718-9 (pbk)
ISBN: 978-0-595-60814-0 (ebk)

Printed in the United States of America

To my daughter Tania, with all my love and my daughter Renee, who too often was in the background because of her sister's brain injury.

Every year 1.4 million Americans sustain a traumatic brain injury. The number of these injuries resulting in lifelong impairment is around 80,000 to 90,000. My daughter Tania is one of these statistics.

CONTENTS

PART THREE: RESOURCES

Preface

I wrote this book to help other families who have a child with a traumatic brain injury. My daughter Tania was thirteen when she was involved in an automobile accident in 1986. She suffered a traumatic brain injury, the severity of which changed her life and the lives of her family forever. During the time of her accident and subsequent treatment and recovery, I found the professional systems around us to be lacking in empathy and support. While the technical medical expertise to keep Tania alive was available, there seemed to be a shortage of awareness for the family's pain, helplessness, and frustration. In addition, information and resources that could have helped us learn and cope were either not available or not easily accessible.

My own journey through this process was like having all sense of control and choice taken from me without my consent. My whole life and identity changed the instant my daughter was injured. At that point, I had ceased being Mary and had become only and completely a mother consumed with the condition of her child. For many months, my own needs and desires disappeared into a fog that cleared only enough to see Tania and nothing else. At the time, the loss of my "self" seemed a small price to pay; however, it ultimately did not serve Tania nor change any of the circumstances in which I found myself.

In addition to grossly neglecting my own needs, the overwhelming stress and grief led to division and conflict within my family. This unhappy side effect of Tania's injury was not unique to us; it was, and is, a frequent occurrence in many families undergoing a similar crisis. It is ironic that just when the family needs to unite and support one another, stress, conflict and denial can drive a wedge between people. One of the reasons this occurs is because family members may be at different stages of denial, grief, or recovery and each is coping in his or her own fashion.

Writing this book first occurred to me when I was working on my Ph.D. in clinical psychology a few years after the accident. My dissertation was "The Mother's Experience of Her Child's Traumatic Brain Injury." I chose this subject because it was foremost in my mind, and I hoped that the information I gained could help both families and the medical community.

In doing my research and writing this book, I used "traumatic brain injury" and "brain injury" to describe both open and closed head injuries. With an open injury, the skull is perforated or penetrated, such as with a gunshot wound. When a closed head injury occurs, the skull remains intact; however, the brain's position shifts, often repeatedly, because of the impact. Common causes of a closed head injury are motor vehicle accidents and falls in which there is an impact on the skull.

While medical technology has greatly advanced to save the lives of children with traumatic brain injuries, the medical community has not caught up to provide the resources and support necessary to help the families deal with the day-to-day situations they face.

My research focused on mothers but certainly fathers experience the same emotions and needs, although fathers might cope somewhat differently with these emotions and needs. It is also important to acknowledge that over the last twenty years, the roles in families have changed. The traditional roles are more blended today than they were when my family initially began to deal with my daughter's injury in 1986. However, mothers are often the primary caregivers and inundated with overwhelming responsibilities that they impose upon themselves. The injured child and the rest of the family's needs frequently come first. Often mothers become so stressed and frazzled, they cannot begin to think about how to carve out some time for their own respite. The mothers and families need to understand that maintaining high levels of stress over time compromises the immune system and makes people more susceptible to illness and disease.

In researching the subject, I called on my own experience and interviewed other mothers who had children with traumatic brain injuries. I found my perceptions validated in my discussions with them. From the interviews, I identified four issues that were common to the experience:

- Emotional and Grieving Issues

- Stress Issues

- Quest for Spiritual Understanding Issues

- Perception of Insufficient Support from the Professional Community Issues

When I was going through the early stages of this ordeal, I wish someone had told me that a brain injury is a process and for many, it is a continuing and evolving process. The injured continue to change and improve throughout their lives; maybe not as dramatically or as quickly as we wish, but there are changes. Even today, after twenty years with Tania's injury, we notice things that let us know she is still improving. Because this recovery is always in flux, families need to be vigilant and innovative in seeking new therapies and techniques for improvement. The medical community is often not aware of things that could help individuals based on their injury, disability, needs, and preferences. With that in mind, it is imperative that families be proactive in seeking information and solutions.

As part of my own personal recovery, I found that I wanted to write not only about my experience with my daughter, but I wanted to share this experience with others. I realized, through the interviews with other mothers, that I could give some value to my ordeal through analyzing, sharing, and offering suggestions to families about how to cope with the situations that arise. Also, I hoped the medical community could gain insight into the emotional needs of families and perhaps develop and implement more effective support systems and resources.

Consequently, I wrote this book to offer hope and knowledge to families with a child afflicted with a traumatic brain injury. Our individual stories may be different, but I am sure we have much in common. Here is how I hope this book can help you:

- Part One is the story of Tania's accident, rehabilitation, and ensuing years to the present date. This will give you an insight and understanding of my journey.

- Part Two gives more details on the issues so many of us face and some of the solutions that may be available to help you.

- Part Three is a resource listing of the most helpful books and Web sites available. I've sifted through thousands of options and selected those I believe most helpful to a family with a child with a traumatic brain injury.

When I think of my experience as a mother of a traumatically brain-injured child, despite the sadness I feel, I realize that this experience also reflects an opening, like a flower in the initial states of blooming. I can take this seemingly worthless experience and create some meaning by helping families and professionals better deal with the trauma.

Mary Burgess-Smith
February 11, 2008

Acknowledgments

I had several wonderful people help me during this journey of writing my book, and I would like to take a moment to thank them:

To Sherrie Arnoldy: thank you for your succinct editing help.

To Peg Campbell: thank you for being with me every step of the book writing experience.

To Linda Detheridge: thank you for your assistance in editing and making the story flow.

To Jeannie Nelson: thank you for your proofreading help.

To Stephen McMath: thank you for the cover artwork.

And especially to my husband Chuck whose loving patience made this journey possible.

Introduction: The Child I Knew

It hurts so much that it is beyond hurt
Where do I start?
These were the words
I wrote to you
A few months
And many light years
Since that early spring eve
That rainy eve
Bringing the promise of spring flowers
This was a cruel storm
Destroying the promise of spring ever since

You were like a flower
Your teens were unfolding
Never to be realized
I often felt like a gardener
With you
Nurturing
Hoping
Proud
It seems all to naught
I love you

At thirteen, my daughter Tania, whom we always called "T", liked listening to loud music, getting together with girlfriends, talking to boys on the telephone for hours, sneaking dirty books under her bed, and getting up for school only an hour before she had to be there. Heaven help anyone who needed the bathroom when she was getting ready. In other words, she was a normal, healthy adolescent.

In school, T was an honor student and worked as a teaching assistant. She enjoyed most sports and was involved in gymnastics and softball. Outside school, she was fond of animals and planned to go to veterinary school. She even designed her own veterinarian clinic. She knew what she wanted, liked to win, and usually did. When she didn't win, she put it behind her and shed very few tears over it.

She was inner-directed and often didn't share her thoughts with me. For instance, we took our new dog to obedience school hoping she would become an indoor dog. When T entered the room with Duchess, the dog immediately bit the trainer. T ran from the room crying. I imagine she felt defeated, but she did not talk about it. We returned the dog to the previous owner, and she never mentioned it again.

One time our cat Lovey was caught in the dryer, and I yelled, "T, Lovey's in the dryer". I was afraid to confront the situation, but T came and opened the dryer door. We immediately took Lovey to the vet and surprisingly she was fine. I was a wreck over the poor creature, but T remained calm and collected. What a role-reversal since I was supposed to be the adult. I was always more sensitive than T, it was as if she came from a different mold. In some ways, T was more like her father: a very directed, take-charge person. Another time, Lovey got sick and had to stay at the vet's office overnight. The vet called me at work to recommend putting the cat to sleep. When I got home, T was sitting on the curb, and I knew that she knew. When we went to the vet to say goodbye to Lovey, I was the one who ran back twice in tears. Finally, T put her arms around me and counseled, "Mom, Lovey is peaceful now." She possessed such wisdom at an early age.

T was always a bubbly child with lots of close friends. Her spontaneous personality drew them in. There were times I thought our personalities did not mesh. I felt I was much more introspective. T was the extrovert who was happy and pleased with things, whatever they were. She was always coming up with ideas and directed people with what to do. Sometimes I think she was on the border of being "bossy." Now I shudder to think of the times I asked her to be quiet so that I could think.

I remember the day I learned I was pregnant with T, and I dragged my husband to a department store to buy a crib. When she was born, I lay in the hospital bed feeling such a bond with her. I remember thinking, "This bond will always hold." And it has, only not in the way I originally hoped. I had thirteen years with her. Do any of my words depict my T? Perhaps, in some way, my words depict her essence, but T was like quick silver and could never be captured. I have internalized this reflection, and it is now part of me.

PART ONE:
THE JOURNEY

CHAPTER 1:
NOT JUST A SPRAINED
ANKLE

On April 1, 1986, my daughter Tania and her friends Heather and Lee were returning from a gymnastics practice. Lee's mother was driving; Lee was in the passenger seat, and Tania and Heather were in the back. At the same time, a 15-year old girl had stolen a car and was being pursued by her brother in a 60 mile-per-hour chase. The driver of the stolen vehicle ran a red light and struck the car in which Tania was riding broadside, with the brunt of the impact to the rear passengers.

It was a rainy Wednesday, and I was glad to be home. Like any working mother with a teenager and a husband to care for, my schedule was a hectic one. I was grateful to Lee's mother for picking up the girls from gymnastics that day because I had a lot to do that evening and didn't want to play chauffeur. When the phone rang, I was loading the dishwasher so Dick took the call. My initial reaction to what Dick was saying was that T had sprained her ankle in gymnastics. I sighed and thought *"Great. Now we have to spend the whole evening sitting around the emergency room, and they'll take an x-ray, wrap the ankle, and send us home with an ice pack at midnight. Just great."* Then I heard Dick say, "You're taking her to University Hospital?" I dropped the plate I was holding. University Hospital was 45 minutes away, and no one would take T there for a sprained ankle. The process of shock and denial protects our psyche when emotions are too intense to bear. After dropping the plate, this numbness set in and insulated me. There was no screaming. There were no tears. There were no bargains with God. It was rare for emotions to seep through this veil. I left the broken plate and went to get my purse with Dick close behind. As we were leaving, we practically bumped into two police officers as they knocked on our door. My heart went to my throat when I saw them. Any news brought personally by police could not be good. The officers asked if we knew there had been an accident, and Dick and I told them we were on our way. We rushed out without stopping for details.

During the ride to the hospital, I watched the wipers swish back and forth in recrimination. I should have been driving my daughter that day. I shouldn't have groused about a sprained ankle for crying out loud. I should have, I should have, I should have … the wipers beat out a rhythm of guilt, and I didn't even know yet what was going on.

Our car pulled into the parking lot as an ambulance arrived. "It's probably T," Dick said. He drove slowly, and I peered out of the window. I was not sure. "It could be any ambulance," I said. Then I saw a wisp of blonde hair on the stretcher, illuminated by the lights at the door, and I knew in an instant it was my T. I sprang from the car and ran to her. Someone held me back. I have been running to catch her ever since.

In the hospital, we were sent to a quiet, pleasantly decorated private room with a phone. I looked around. *This is the Serious Room. This is the room where they hide the families who might receive the worst possible news. This is where they put the screamers and weepers so the regular folks with sprained ankles and such might not see them and get frightened away* … Someone offered us coffee. We were joined by Heather's parents and the school principal, who had assisted the authorities in identifying the girls and notifying the families. Heather, who was sitting next to T in the car, was also injured. Heather's parents, Dick, and I sat tight in the Serious Room, bound by concern and apprehension as we tried to piece together what had happened to our children. We knew that all four occupants of the vehicle had been injured and were currently being treated in the Emergency Room. We knew that the front passengers, Lee and her mother, experienced fewer traumas than our girls but aside from that, information was scarce and slow in coming.

As the hours ticked by, I could not keep my mind from T. I kept thinking of T being alone in there, imagining her frightened and lost without me. I tried repeatedly to be with her, but they would not allow me in. I looked at the paintings on the wall until I had memorized them. I studied the upholstery on the couch thread by thread. I became intimately acquainted with a certain spot on the rug until I knew it like an old friend. I waited and did not act upon my desire to run screaming from the Serious Room and tackle my way to my little girl's side.

Finally, we were notified that T and Heather had both been transferred to the ICU. The nurse told Dick and me that we should not go in since they hadn't yet had a chance to clean T up. She suggested we go home and get some rest, as if that were possible. I protested. This woman must be out of her mind. How would she feel in my place? Would she leave her daughter? Dick shushed me and said that it may be a good idea. I could only stare at him, feeling as if my support had crumbled at my feet, but I allowed him to take us home to face the familiar, which now seemed a thousand miles away.

When we got to the house in the early morning, I walked into the living room, picked up Tania's school picture, and began to cry. Dick tried to comfort me by saying, "We don't know how bad it is." I knew it was bad enough. The veil settled back into place. I felt dejected but non-emotional. This feeling of dejection lasted some time. Dick went to sleep with an ease that I both envied and resented. Whatever pain he felt was wrapped up tight inside him, and I was alone in my grief. I sat, much as I had in the hospital, kicking myself for leaving. My baby was hurt, and I had walked away. What if she was, at this very moment, asking for me? I wept and wandered through the house with a sorrow so deep it seemed bottomless.

We returned to the hospital ICU the next morning, but no doctors were around to talk with us about T's condition. I went into the room and found her hooked to a mass of wires and tubes. Her swollen face had lacerations, her front teeth were knocked out, and she had a broken arm and leg. She didn't move. It wasn't evident that she was in any pain, but that was little comfort. Just yesterday, T had been chatting and laughing and gossiping like any other healthy teenager. Now she was wounded and broken and whatever pain she was spared, I took inside myself. I would have taken all of it, gladly, to have her be intact again. T looked peaceful, though, and I took hope from that. *She'll wake up, and she'll be fine. The cuts will heal, and the bones will mend. The teeth can be fixed. We'll go on, and she'll return to school. It's not so bad … it's not so bad … it's not so bad.*

Dick had left his wallet at the house and had gone home to retrieve it. I was alone with T when a neurosurgeon entered the room with a CT scan in her hand. She told me her name, which meant nothing to me, then abruptly informed me that T had less than a 1 percent chance to live and even less of a chance to wake up. The doctor delivered this news without a kind word and exited the room in a flurry of white coat and bustle, unable or unwilling to watch me try to catch this information and struggle with its weight. The doctor didn't see the blood leave my face. She didn't see me lose my balance and stumble backward. She didn't see the nurse catch me and sit me down. The doctor had run from this to continue on her rounds, or go to lunch, or cash her check. I was left drowning in her wake, like someone who had fallen off a ship only to watch it sail away.

When my other daughter Renee arrived at the hospital from Michigan State University where she was going to school, I told her what the neurosurgeon said and complained of her hasty manner. Renee was so disturbed by this that she went to talk to the administrators in the neurosurgery department. To this day, I have a hard time thinking about that morning without feeling some resentment toward the neurosurgeon for acting so uncaring and cold.

When Dick returned, we were faced with making an immediate major decision. Another neurosurgeon said T could be placed in a deeper barbiturate coma to relieve the pressure on her brain caused by the swelling. However, this procedure would decrease the likelihood that T would live through the night. He asked what we wanted to do. I was thinking about funerals and could not make a decision. How could I make a choice like that? Dick's immediate response was, "Let's go for it." Then I agreed; it was almost like we had nothing to lose.

That evening found us in the hospital chapel with Renee and her friend, my parents, and their minister. We did not attend church regularly, but my Lutheran parents did. In the small chapel, I found myself asking, "Why" over and over again. In answer, the minister said that God has a plan for T that we were unable to figure out. That was not a satisfactory explanation for me and made me feel extremely frustrated with the minister and his God. On the other hand, Dick decided he wanted T baptized and so the minister performed that ritual.

Even though we weren't far from home, we decided to get a room at the hospital's hotel, the Med Inn, for a couple of days. It would give us a place to sleep as well as a place to escape to when keeping a vigil in T's room was too exhausting. We slept at the Med Inn that night and the next morning found T's condition unchanged. She was still alive, and I was ecstatic. I felt a surge of hope. Bonnie, the ICU nurse, said, "You know this does not change anything." Her words could not penetrate the euphoria in my mind and held very little meaning for me. In retrospect, I see this was my first encounter with denial. My denial buoyed me up until the abrupt neurosurgeon from Hell breezed in with the results of the CT scans. She told us T would probably never wake up; and if she did, we would wish she had not. The surgeon delivered this news with a generous helping of indifference covered in ice. In a way, I was grateful for her lack of compassion. The fantasy I had of grabbing her by her starched, white collar and flinging her out the window gave me a focal point for my anger and grief, which were danger-ously close to consuming me.

The University Hospital is a grand and glorious machine. When a patient such as T is admitted to the ICU, some mechanism goes into operation deep in the bowels of the place, and social workers are dispensed like artificially sweet-ened candy. While I appreciated the intentions of these well-meaning people who visited with my daughter's file tucked neatly under their arms, I found them mostly intrusive. They simply would not leave us alone, and the questions they asked were not helpful but actually quite irritating. Although the social workers were well-trained and competent in their field, it just seemed to us that they had no clue about what we really needed. For that matter, we didn't know what we really needed ourselves. Most of the time, we just wanted to be left alone to feel and say what occurred to us as each moment passed without being observed, ana-lyzed, or advised.

For example, a social worker in the ICU said to me, "You're not crying." I was puzzled because I spent most of the night crying. Was I not living up to some social worker quota of tears? Was I being categorized by this veritable stranger as some kind of inefficient griever? Was I supposed to cry all the time? As it was, I could barely see; my eyes were so swollen and sore. All I could do was stare at this woman and wonder if she had ever actually felt any of the emotions she was to monitor.

Apparently, I had not satisfied the social workers' appetites for disclosure, so they turned to Renee. One social worker asked her if she was close to her sister. Although the social worker may have been looking for a way to lead into a con-versation with her, in reality Renee found this question quite invasive. "I do not want to discuss my relationship with my sister with anyone," she said so that everyone could hear. I was proud of her for standing her own emotional ground, but I suspected Renee avoided the question in part because she and T hadn't been particularly close. Renee had been an only child for the seven years before T was born, so the gap in their ages meant they didn't have much in common. Renee was much more quiet and introspective than T. She was usually soft-spo-ken, and I always felt she was much more like me. Both of us are easy to get along with but if we feel strongly about something, we will go after it in a directed, determined way. T was more like her father: a take-charge person to the point of being domineering. I remember when T was in kindergarten and I arrived to pick her up. She had several of her classmates sitting in a row while she was teaching them something. Renee would have never done anything like that. At the hospital, however, Renee displayed her own will in a fashion that would have rivaled T's.

There was one person who did help us and that was Julie, the hospital chaplain. Julie simply sat with us and talked if we wanted to or remained silent. She also stopped by to visit and talk to T if we were not there. It was a great comfort to have Chaplain Julie on our team; I felt she was there for me as well as for T.

The nurses told us that hearing is the last thing to go and perhaps T could hear us talking and even recognize our voices. We tried to keep some auditory stimulation going for her by either talking to her or having her favorite music playing in the background just in case. In addition, we kept a notebook by T's bed to write the things about which we were chatting with her. Conversations were mostly concerning her cats and general things going on. Many times I would pick up that notebook and read the early morning writings by Julie. We had brought T her favorite music, and Julie always made sure it was on in the background. Talking to T and playing her music made us feel like we were doing something for her. I also manicured and polished her fingernails and made sure she always looked pretty, but it was not enough because it didn't cure her. It was what I could do to nurture her, yet it was so little. No matter what I did for her, I always felt as if I had let her down. I hadn't protected her, and I could never change that.

Dick returned to work, and Renee returned to campus. We kept our room at the Med Inn, and it became a welcome relief from the vigil I was keeping at T's bedside. We visited our home periodically to check on the cats. I felt as if I was functioning on a different plane from the rest of the world. I had dug a trench between a hotel room and a hospital room, and I was beginning to feel as if I had walked that trench for years. In a matter of days, the world I knew before T's accident felt like someone else's memory.

Although I did my best to hold my emotions in check most of the time, they would swoop up and surprise me like snipers. Grief would come out of nowhere and ambush me. Once, I walked into T's room at home and found a half-eaten package of gummy bears. She had left it, I imagine, where she might pick it up and finish it later. T wouldn't get to those gummy bears for a very long time, if ever. The sight of that abandoned bit of candy struck me right in my gut and caused me to double over in tears. Dick, on the other hand, appeared to go on with his life. Perhaps his way of coping was simply to throw himself into his daily routine but without evidence that he was feeling what I felt; I was lonely and isolated.

T's friend Heather was still in a coma as well, and her mother and I spent many hours sitting together hoping our daughters would wake up. (Heather, by the way, stayed in a coma for about two months, and then woke up and started therapy. While she did recover somewhat, she still has brain damage and exhibits learning disabilities.) Some of the girls' friends from school would come to visit but that quickly ended because for them, nothing was gratifying about the visit and, in fact, it was very traumatic for them to see their unconscious classmates. T's best friend Danielle had witnessed the car crash on her way home from gymnastics that night. She came to the hospital to visit, but she was so traumatized by the experience that her mother made her stop visiting.

Thinking back to those first few days and weeks, I remember the exhaustion of sitting by T's bed for hours, holding her hand, talking to her, playing music for her, and hoping. I was doing all this and there was no way of knowing if she even knew I was there, or even who I was. There were days I washed my hair repeatedly. There were days I cried for hours. There were many days I couldn't remember if I had eaten or simply forgot to feed myself all together. In hindsight, I realize that I was in the initial stage of the grieving process, commonly referred to as denial. The denial process is a coping or defense mechanism that helps people adjust to extreme situations by denying their severity or existence. In my own case, I didn't listen to nor did I internalize the dire prognosis the doctors pronounced. I believed that at any moment, my little girl would awaken and everything would be back to normal. When the staff handed me pamphlets from the Michigan Head Injury Alliance, which probably would have been helpful at the time, I just put them away without reading them. I couldn't understand how they pertained to me. It was classic denial, I know now.

After two months, T was transferred out of the ICU to the rehabilitation unit. During the days and nights of being by T's side, I began to wish for a place of refuge. Being with T so much was beginning to make me wish I had a place to go, just to get away from the hole I was stuck in at the hospital. Then I remembered meditation. Before the accident, I had been studying Zen and learned that there was a center in Ann Arbor. The Zen Center was only a few blocks from the hospital, and it was there that I found a sanctuary. I was grateful to experience a sense of serenity at the Zen Center. The director's name was Sukha, and she, like Julie, became a source of comfort and support for me. The Zen Center was very quiet in contrast to the hustle and bustle at University Hospital. At the Zen Center, if people spoke at all it was in quiet tones. The meditation allowed a gentle turning inward and gave me the ability to let thoughts go.

It took me a long time to realize that I lost the daughter I had known and loved for thirteen years. Although she didn't die in the car crash that rainy night, the child who emerged on the other side of time barely resembles that energetic thirteen-year-old girl who ran off to gymnastics that fateful day. I feel as if a part of her and a part of me also died in the car crash that night. This is part of a unique grieving process where the lost person still lives.

I remember one Zen sitting on a particularly hot day. We usually drank hot tea and during a break from meditation, Sukha brought ice for my tea. This may not seem like much by itself, but in the order of the Zen discipline, it is quite noteworthy. Zen is about being humble, not complaining, and accepting things for the way they are. I found the fact that Sukha brought me ice on this hot day extraordinarily touching and kind. I asked Sukha once about T's accident in my continuing quest for a reason. Sukha replied simply that she had seen a squirrel hit by a car that morning, and a flower she had nurtured died. I took this to mean that change is an inevitable part of life, in accordance with Zen philosophy. Despite my intellectual understanding of this, I still ached for a sense of purpose to the tragedy that had befallen my daughter and my family. In another conversation with Sukha about my prayers and meditation practice; she said "Tania is your practice". She has become in many ways my way of being in this world.

Chapter 2:
Trying to cope

I had actually returned to work two weeks after the accident because T was still in a coma, and I realized that spending all my days at the hospital was not helpful to anyone. I was becoming depressed at the hospital and since Dick was working and Renee was back in school, I was alone there most of the time. T's prognosis had not changed, and it didn't seem as if I was making a difference. Working was a diversion for me and helped me focus on something other than T.

I taught in the child psychology unit at a local hospital. Part of my job was to evaluate children academically when they were admitted, develop a lesson plan so that they would not fall behind while being hospitalized, and make recommendations to their school upon their discharge. The other part of my job was in a team-teaching role, and my partner Cliff and I dealt with adolescents. Unfortunately, Cliff had to rely on nursing personnel to help during my absence because our teaching staff did not take into account people not being there in situations such as mine. On the first afternoon I was back, I walked into the class and the kids were pretty much out of control, running and yelling around the room and being anything but model students. Cliff was just letting them go, and it was pretty evident that he had lost all control. Cliff's philosophy was, "The pay's good … don't rock the boat." When he saw me, he shrugged and said, "These are the kids we have now."

In this setting, children stayed hospitalized until their insurance ran out which was about six weeks. It was a revolving door with students coming and going daily. The area the hospital drew from was inner city Detroit, so we had some pretty street-wise kids. The person who filled in while I was gone was from the nursing staff, not really a teacher, and coped with the chaos by yelling at the students and threatening to pull their evening TV privileges. While it kept them in line, it wasn't an optimal learning situation. I had my work cut out for me, and I was grateful for a problem outside of my own on which to focus.

Within the classroom, there was so much to do that there were actually times I didn't think about T. Outside our classroom, however, I felt my coworkers did not know how to respond to me. I was not much help to them because I actually wanted to be left alone. People would try to be polite in inquiring about T, but the truth is I found myself repeating the same story over and over. This forced me to think about T. Even worse, it forced me to think about the fact that I had not been thinking about her. Perhaps sensing my discomfort, my coworkers treated me with kid gloves, as though I might fragment at any moment like a piece of cracked glass. Everyone at the school was very nice to me, and people I never talked with before the accident were now coming up to me and talking. At times, I felt that their concern might not be genuine. I didn't have much to do outside of the classroom because my coworkers assumed most of my administrative duties. I understood they were only trying to help, but I actually would have preferred to have something more to do.

The staff tried hard to be supportive in many ways. They organized a drive to collect blood in case T needed it. One of the head psychologists gave Dick and me tickets for a symphony. He thought we needed to do something fun together. We did go to the symphony, but it seemed surreal. I felt as if I should have been at the hospital and could not enjoy the beautiful music because my mind kept going to the events in our lives.

When I was not teaching, I was at the hospital holding T's hand. I continued telling her about her cats and the world around her, not knowing if she could even hear me. I functioned, but I was both physically and emotionally exhausted. We lived thirty miles from University Hospital, and it was another ten miles in the other direction to my school. After a couple weeks of commuting from school to the hospital and then home, I realized it would greatly relieve my stress if I taught part-time. I filed a request for part-time status in order to be with T more. The administration told me they could not change the status of the job. I don't even remember if they gave me a reason, but I returned with a letter from my doctor requesting the status be changed to decrease my stress level. I sent a copy to Human Relations, and the status magically changed. Reduction in the time I spent teaching helped alleviate some of the stress I was feeling and made it easier for me to deal with the situation.

During this time, I held onto my hope for T's recovery like a lifeline. With all the knowledge the medical profession possesses about the human brain, they did not have a way to project what would happen. The human brain seemed to be as mysterious to the experts as it was to me, and miracles happened every day when it appeared hope was lost. I held my hope close to my heart, like a precious secret. Was this denial to have hope? Hope and denial traveled hand-in-hand, and I left the door open to both. I did not allow information to the contrary of hope enter my consciousness. Hope exists in an uncertain outcome. I did not assume T would be like she was before the accident or that she would even be independent. I simply hoped she would wake up and be in a state where she could have some quality to her life. One of the resident physicians treating T was very sympathetic and told me that this was "the worst thing that can happen to a parent." He continued to say that at some point the abnormal would become normal. My only thought at the time was that he had no idea what he was talking about but later his words came back to me again and again.

T continued to consume my whole life. When I was home alone, I would listen to a tape T and her friend Jenny had made in Arizona. I kept playing it so I would not forget the sound of her voice. I loved listening to their flip way of talking about boys, clothes, movies, and more boys. According to T and Jenny, it was all just so "cool." T and Jenny made the tape a couple of years before when T, Renee, and I moved to Arizona. Dick and I had been struggling with some marital issues, and I thought a separation might help us determine what we ought to do next.

T loved it in Arizona from the moment we arrived. She ran around the apartment complex, investigating things, and expressing delight in the whirlpool. After her first day of school, I picked her up and talked with her teacher, Mrs. Tomleson. It turned out that she was one of the best teachers I have ever met. Mrs. Tomleson told me T stood in front of the class, introduced herself, and proudly announced, "I am from Michigan." She quickly made many new friends.

Renee had a harder time adjusting. She was a senior in high school and not happy about attending a new school. In addition, the small town in which we lived was stifling to her. Las Vegas was ninety miles away, and we had to go there to do any significant shopping. I was greatly relieved when she found a "best friend" and then started dating. She began to blossom like a southwestern desert flower and is still in contact with her girl friend.

Dick and I spoke on the phone almost daily, and he visited us regularly. Our situation seemed more like a long-distance romance than a separation. At the end of the school year, the girls and I returned to Michigan, considerably more tanned and more centered.

Listening to the tape of T reminded me how resilient she had always been, jumping into new situations with no hesitation. I felt comfort in listening to their voices and the way they liked to exaggerate words with a lot of inflection in their voices.

T's voice sometimes came to me in my dreams. Several months after the accident, I had a dream about T in which I was attempting to process all that had happened after the accident. T said in that somewhat flip voice of hers, "What is all the fuss about?" This was a reflection of how she could face dreadful situations with a matter-of-factness that I did not possess. If she had been able, I knew that she would have guided me through this crisis with grace and control. It was ironic that I needed her so much to help me and now she was so helpless and out of reach.

I did the best I could to think like T and do what she would have wanted. In the rehab unit, the nurses wanted to simulate a "normal" life and wanted the patients to start feeling less like patients. The staff dressed them in their own clothes such as T-shirts and shorts rather than hospital gowns. I continued to make sure T looked nice. I painted her fingernails and toenails, brushed her hair, and pulled it back with barrettes. I dabbed her favorite perfume behind her ears hoping the scent would get through to her. Although wearing her own clothes made the situation seem less institutional, it did not change the fact that T was in a coma. It really made no difference what she wore or how pretty she looked.

We had the choice of whether T's laundry was done in the hospital or at home. I preferred to do it because it made me feel like I was doing something for her. Like fixing her hair and nails, washing T's clothes helped me but did nothing for her. I felt so powerless; I was powerless. Moms are supposed to be able to fix anything. We kiss the boo-boos and protect our children at all costs. There is an agony and despair when your child is hurt that tugs at a mother's soul. I cried beyond my capacity to cry, always amazed that I had tears left. They stayed with me for such a long time.

My sense of time was altered. One of the rescue team members said the accident lasted one and a half seconds. Sometimes it seems the accident happened a long time ago, while other times it feels as recent as last night's dream. However, I do not wake up. Some call it the endless nightmare. It often feels like a state of animated suspension with an overwhelming feeling of helplessness.

Chapter 3:
Transfer to Virginia

In September, five months after the accident, the University of Michigan Hospital staff wanted to discharge T from the hospital because she had not progressed enough. She was unresponsive to her environment. When they transferred her to the rehabilitation floor months earlier, the hope was that she would wake up. T continued in the coma and was taking up valuable room in an environment that could do nothing more for her. Consequently, they suggested she be moved to a nursing home, with rehabilitation as an option if she woke up. All our family members were experiencing the frustration of feeling as if there was no help from the medical staff or services to support the family.

I could not imagine putting T in a facility generally thought to be for old and feeble people. It seemed like the last stop before hopelessness and death; a place where she would be maintained and slowly forgotten. All I could think was, "I'll show them … she'll wake up." I would sit by her bed willing her to open her eyes. Dick's mother also resisted the idea. Although she usually stayed in the background, she spoke out vehemently against the transfer saying, "There is no way my granddaughter is going into a nursing home." I was proud of her and considered her my ally in the debate. Although we understood the hospital's position, we simply did not know where to go from there. We examined all the rehabilitation facilities in Michigan. None of them seemed appropriate. We felt pushed by the hospital to leave, but they offered little or no assistance in locating an alternative for T. Finding proper rehabilitation facilities only added to my stress and to the stress of the family. We seemed to have few choices.

Then we found a brochure for a facility in Virginia. It explained how they responded to the complex needs of brain-injured patients. It highlighted their skilled clinicians who had built a comprehensive array of services for patients with traumatic brain injuries, from coma-recovery to comprehensive acute rehabilitation, as well as sub-acute and longer-term sub-acute rehabilitation. It said they treated patients from all over the country. It sounded like just what we needed, so we contacted them and a representative from their pediatric unit came to University Hospital to meet us and perform an assessment on T. The representative was extremely positive. That was so refreshing because everything we had been hearing was pessimistic. She had glossy brochures and a video of kids in rehab running around. The facility looked like a spa with its manicured grounds and acres of woods and natural lakes. If we had been in the right frame of mind, Dick and I would have visited the facility but because we didn't want to put T in a nursing home and felt pressured to move her, we decided to transfer her to the Virginia facility based solely on pictures and the presentation made by the representative.

I took vacation time from my job so I could fly with T to the new facility. She was transferred in a med-evac unit, which is a medically equipped aircraft. She wore a new outfit I gave her for her birthday, and I felt an unrealistic sense of pride as if she were off to her first day of school. I had high hopes that this new facility with its specialized staff would be just the thing T needed for recovery. When I arrived with T and looked around at the grounds and buildings, I was extremely impressed with their beauty, and my hopes seemed justified. My feelings quickly changed, however, when I talked to the doctor in charge. He told me that T would probably be staying only a few months. The staff wanted only "Success Stories", and she did not fit the profile of patients they wanted. I had hoped that when they tested her they would find some improvement because I thought the coma had lessened. I had been with T so much that I was aware of subtle changes, and I was sure she was moving toward consciousness. It saddened me deeply when they placed a small golden kitten on her bed and she failed to respond. Cats have always been her favorite animal, and I was devastated that she had no reaction. I realize now that my expectations were probably unrealistic. I was so hoping that the medical experts would validate my perceptions, but they did not. Their opinion was that T was not progressing. I was extremely disappointed and angry after the conversation with the doctor in charge. When I thought about all the trouble we went through to transfer T, and how positive the representative had been, I burned with anger. Now I was told that not only would her stay be short, but this wonderful, specialized facility could not offer any hope to help her as well.

Although the facility was only an hour from Richmond, it seemed to be in the middle of nowhere. I did not have a car, and Dick would not arrive until the weekend. I spent my time with T. I dwelled on how unnecessary this move actually may have been if they wanted to transfer her out because she would not be one of their success stories. How dare they reject my daughter because of public relations. I felt betrayed on a fundamental level, and a bit like a sucker who had bought a phony elixir. I called Dick and had a very teary conversation with him. He suggested we begin looking for another facility right away.

The next days until Dick arrived were sad and lonely. Fortunately, there was an extremely charming housing setup for parents. It was warm and cozy. It reminded me of southern hospitality with soft chairs, sofas, and gentle lighting from charming little lamps. It was almost possible to forget why I was there in this homey environment. Under other circumstances, it would have been a lovely, serene retreat.

When Dick arrived, we visited with T and then went out for dinner. I got teary-eyed as soon as we sat down. I told Dick again about the disappointing conversation with the doctor. Dick did not react like me and simply said, "We'll have to see where we can go from here." That was Dick, so matter of fact and logical about everything. That was how his brain worked. I think it was a by-product of his engineering education, or engineering was a by-product of his way of thinking. He didn't even comment on how attractive the grounds were or the beauty of the surrounding lush woods and natural lakes. Although this was the man with whom I shared my life, I couldn't help but wish for some sign, any sign, that he felt as deeply as I about our situation. This difference between us, though most certainly a difference in coping styles, caused me to feel disconnected from my husband. Intellectually, I probably understood that Dick was just being Dick, but emotionally how I ached to resonate with him. I flew home with Dick at the end of the weekend, wondering if he felt as horrible as I for leaving T behind or if he felt relief. I never knew.

Our insurance company financed two trips a month to Virginia. We would fly in on a Friday night, get in after 9:00 PM, and make a stop at the facility to check in on T. At that time of day, the evening crew was on duty and they had very little information about T's progress. In fact, no one on the night staff ever had anything concrete to tell us. Each time I left Michigan on Friday, I would hope that I would arrive in Virginia to find T awake. We spent the weekends with T, who was unresponsive. Our only outlet on these weekends was going out to dinner. Actually, the whole experience was dismal.

Again, I was on the roller coaster ride. There were dizzying heights of hope one minute and deep valleys of despair the next. The direction up or down depended on which doctor I talked to at the time. I searched for any glimmer of hope I could find and was constantly interpreting anything except the most negative news as a positive. I read whatever I could find about brain injury and comas. I became very familiar with the Rancho Los Amigos Scale. It is helpful in assessing the patient in the first weeks or months following a brain injury because it does not require cooperation from the patient. The scale relies on observations of the patient's response to external stimuli. It provides a descriptive guideline of the eight stages a brain injury patient will experience as they progress through recovery (Mitiguy, Thompson, & Wasco 1990).

According to the Rancho Los Amigos Scale, I figured T would be rated a Stage Four. Stage Four patients experience purposeless agitation with a heightened state of activity. I noted on my visits to Virginia that T was moving around for the first time with seemingly little purpose. When I suggested to the doctor that T might be somewhere in the middle of the Scale, he disagreed. He said she was definitely not a Stage Four patient and was really showing no progress at all.

Dick's mother came out to visit when T had been in Virginia for a while. My mother-in-law had been as hopeful as I was but at this point, she seemed to give up. She walked out of T's room, obviously upset, and said she did not think T would ever get any better. It had been six months since the accident. I spent some time in Virginia looking around at the rooms where the facility's success stories were receiving rehabilitation. The children's room was loud; there were children crying, screaming, and talking at full volume. Their speech often made very little sense, as they spoke with disjointed and fragmented sentences. I thought, "This is so different from the video the representative had shown us in Michigan." The children in the video were obviously the super success stories, and the video had shown them learning and interacting with the staff and others. I felt deceived because these chaotic rehabilitation rooms were not at all what I had been told to expect.

As we started researching other facilities, I began to feel like my mother-in-law. I was starting to give up on T's recovery and was now looking for a place that would provide her comatose body with optimum care. The Head Injury Alliance in Michigan recommended a rehabilitation facility in New York called Arbordale. Arbordale was part of New Medico, a national health care network which specialized in treating brain injuries. Arbordale was about an hour away from Syracuse. Although I would have preferred to have T back in Michigan, Syracuse was no less inconvenient than Virginia at this point.

Before I even considered moving T again, I wanted to see the facility in person. I wasn't about to make the same mistake of buying into a program based on a dog and pony show from a sales representative. I went to New York without high expectations. As much as I had tried to keep hope for T alive, every physician we had talked to up until that time had the same prognosis: T would not wake up and if she did, we would have wished she had not.

Maybe it was due to my new, realistic attitude, but I was favorably impressed with my visit with Arbordale. The staff was warm and caring. When I met with the medical director, Dr. Barry, he spoke with optimism about T. He had studied her file and expressed hope regarding her condition. I was pleased with what Dr. Barry was saying, but I was steadily giving up on T ever waking up. Everyone else had given up; who was I to disagree?

Around this time, I wrote in my journal "I have lost you, as I know you … You are gone, and you will never be back." I remember thinking, as I wrote, that I could not believe that T once wrote like this. She loved writing, and English was one of her favorite subjects. Now she did not even recognize me. Sometimes I wondered where her thirteen years of knowledge went. How can someone's thoughts and dreams, fears and experiences just vanish? I felt like T's future and mine were a complex jigsaw puzzle with pieces that changed shape and were ill fitting. How could I possibly help heal my daughter when there seemed to be so much that was missing? My baby was fractured; the whole of her had just disappeared.

CHAPTER 4:
TRANSFER TO NEW YORK

After four months at the facility in Virginia, we moved T to New York. When I arrived, I was aware of the contrast between Arbordale's hospital setting and the spa-like Virginia facility. Then I immediately recalled my initial visit here and how warm and caring all the staff had been. Who cared about trees and lakes? The scenery had contributed nothing to my daughter's recovery and had only served to make us feel better about a choice that had ultimately proved wrong.

I met again with Dr. Barry. He reviewed the information on T with me and once again presented a hopeful picture. He said she was moving around in an agitated fashion and was most likely a Stage Four on the Rancho Los Amigos Scale. I should have found some satisfaction in Dr. Barry's confirmation of my own observations, but I had no sense of vindication. I had swung to the Dark Side and now I disregarded the positive as strongly as I had once rejected the negative. After all this time, what was the point? Hope just led to despair, and I had had my fill of despair.

I didn't shut Dr. Barry out completely, however. He had spent time researching the emotional process of families in dealing with a child's head injury. It was comforting to find someone, finally, who had both an interest and an expertise in those of us who were collateral damage. Dr. Barry believes grief is both a reaction to loss and an important aspect of recovery. He broke the grieving process down in stages for me: the first stage is shock and denial. The second stage is anxiety and panic. The third stage is anger, sometimes experienced as guilt. The last stage is one of depression. Dr. Barry told me that in order for families to accept the loss they are experiencing, grief must first occur. He also believed that mourning is a natural part of the grief process. My own mourning over T had been very solitary. Dr. Barry pointed out that in many families members are at different stages of the grieving continuum at any given time. Therefore, each is trying to console another from a very different point of view, which can be confusing, frustrating, and irritating.

Dr. Barry's input was helpful because it offered an explanation for the emotional isolation I had been feeling from my husband and the rest of my family. Dick was obviously in a different place from me, and I could not expect him to have the same reactions. My husband had found a channel for his own grief by focusing on the teenage driver of the car that struck T. The girl had survived the accident, and Dick was far more interested than I in seeing justice prevail. He attended the court proceedings and vented much rage against the teen. Oddly enough, I did not feel anger toward the girl. It was never an issue for me. I understand now that Dick was only finding a way out for his own inner turmoil and though it wasn't my style, our basic emotions were the same.

We maintained the same schedule going to New York as we had when we traveled to Virginia. Every other weekend we would fly in on Friday night, make a late night visit to the facility, and then go on to our hotel. We spent Saturdays talking with T in her comatose state and would go to dinner in the evenings. On Sundays, we would stop by the hospital and then fly home. It was like that old expression, Same S--t, Different State.

When we were back in Michigan, Dick and I began talking about building another house. We had purchased over an acre of wooded property some time earlier with the intent of someday building a home. We knew that if we moved T back to Michigan, our home would need to be handicap accessible with ramps and wide doorways. We thought the timing on building a new house would be workable. We hired an architect and designed a New England style saltbox house. For many people building a house would be a stressful situation but for us, it was an exciting project. Designing and building a new home gave us something on which to focus and take our minds off the fate of T. We built the house on the side of a hill, and it felt like we were living in a tree house, especially on the second floor. We put T's room on the first floor with her own bathroom with safety rails. The new house was what was left of my hope. If we built it, she would come.

CHAPTER 5:
MY MEDICAL SAGA

"… And just when I think I have lost everything, when I do not think I can bear any-more, I find there is still something they can take from me."—*"Out of Africa."*

Shortly after we moved T to New York, I found a lump in my breast that seemed different from the fibrocystic lumps I had experienced in the past. This lump was painful. I had been seeing a surgeon at the University of Michigan Hospital for the fibrocystic problem, and he performed a biopsy. The biopsy was positive, and I was diagnosed with breast cancer. When the surgery was scheduled, all I could think was, "I do not have time for this. I need to be in New York with T."

The evening before surgery, the surgeon met with Dick and me. He was very serious. He said he had spent a lot of time the night before looking at my tests. He knew it was cancer and thought it would be best to remove the whole breast. I was shocked because I assumed they would just remove the lump. I asked how he could be so sure removing the whole breast was necessary. He said he couldn't be one hundred percent sure at this point about how much needed to be removed and where it may have metastasized but based on his experience, he thought removing the whole breast was the prudent thing to do. The impact of what he was saying suddenly hit me. "You mean I am going to go into the operating room and I will come out without a breast?" I asked. He nodded, and I snapped, "How would you like to go in there and come out without a penis?" I looked at Dick. He was visibly shocked by my outburst because it was so unlike me. I guess that made him realize how traumatic this situation was for me. I was usually easy to get along with because, by my nature, I generally agreed with what people said. However, when someone told me something I couldn't accept or didn't agree with, they saw another side of me. Dick was consoling and tried to comfort me. He promised to support me through surgery and reconstruction.

While I was waiting to get my room assignment, I remembered Julie, the chaplain at this hospital, whom we met after T's accident. She had been so comforting then and I wondered if she was still on staff. One of the nurses checked for me and shortly after, Julie appeared and promised to stay with me through surgery. Unfortunately, they couldn't find a hospital bed for me at University Hospital. Bad as the situation was, it was more of an inconvenience compared to all the trauma and distress I had experienced, and having Julie with me made it more tolerable. Finally, they located a vacant bed at the Kellogg Eye Center, which was about three blocks away from the main hospital. By the time I finally got settled in the hospital room, it was 1:00 AM, and Dick went home for the night. Julie stayed with me. I tried to sleep that night, but I couldn't relax. I felt I was just waiting, just waiting. Even though I was dreading the surgery, I was relieved when morning came. Dick returned, and we went over to surgery. Julie sat with Dick until I was in recovery. She is the closest thing to an angel I have found.

After the mastectomy, the doctor prescribed a follow up plan for radiation treatments. Again, my thought was I did not have time for that because I needed to be in New York with T. The more practical side of me prevailed, however, for how could I be there for T if I didn't beat this cancer? I underwent radiation treatments and reconstructive surgery for six weeks after the surgery.

From the outside, it must have appeared that I just breezed through the cancer. Certainly, my concern for T did prove to distract me from my own condition, but I was not immune to fear. Having breast cancer made me realize my own vulnerability and mortality. Once when I was driving home from a radiation treatment, it hit me that what I was going through was serious and that I could actually die from this. Living in that moment, thinking that I could die, made me realize something. I didn't want to die, not only because my family needed me but because I needed me. In the past few months, I had forgotten that there were things I wanted out of my life. There were goals and dreams I had for Mary and although I had put them aside, they had not vanished completely. In the face of my own mortality, I decided that it was time to resurface.

I had always wanted a Ph.D. in clinical psychology. I was going to get it. I talked with Dick about going to graduate school, and he thought it was a great idea. Some of my friends weren't as supportive; they were concerned that I would be taking on too much. I thought of T, who was almost a year into her coma. The medical profession had given up on her waking up, and I had, too. I thought of what T would have said about graduate school. She would have said, "It's cool, Mom. Go for it." So, I did.

Returning to school saved my life. It was a tremendous challenge but ultimately allowed me to grow, return to myself, and regain control. This was important since the main part of my life involving T was so out of control. It was actually ironic that tackling graduate school would greatly increase the stress in most people's lives yet for me, it was a stress outlet.

School was concrete. I felt as if I could actually get my arms around it. It gave me a goal on which to focus and gave me a sense of achievement. At the beginning, the Ph.D. seemed a long way away, but I felt productive and enjoyed the sense of accomplishment as each class ended. Most of all, it was a great creative outlet for me. I had another part to my life, finally. For the first time in a long time, not everything I did revolved around being in the hospital with T.

I enrolled in the Center for Humanistic Studies Graduate School. I had heard wonderful things about this school, and it was fairly close to home. It was a small, professional graduate school specializing in Humanistic and Clinical Psychology. The Center offered a four-year doctoral degree in humanistic and clinical psychology. Humanistic psychology is a contemporary and integrative school of thought committed to affirming the inherent value and dignity of human beings, and this greatly appealed to me. Clark Moustakas was one of the founders of Humanistic and Clinical Psychology in 1956. The publication of his book, The Self, was the impetus for the original dialogues between himself, Abraham Maslow, Carl Rogers, and others, which forged the Humanistic Psychology movement. Meetings were held at 40 East Ferry Avenue in Detroit and later this address became the first home of the Center for Humanistic Studies. Then it moved to Farmington Hills, Michigan, and most recently the school changed its name to the Michigan School of Professional Psychology.

I had some supportive advisors who helped me with my class selections. I had one supervisor who kept an open door policy for me to discuss T or anything else with which I felt I needed assistance. Many faculty members were encouraging. The buildings were reconstructed old homes and the library had overstuffed chairs and couches. It began to feel like a second home to me. The Center for Humanistic Studies was exactly the nurturing environment I needed to heal and grow.

CHAPTER 6:
TANIA WAKES UP

Around Christmas, nine months after the accident, T remained generally unresponsive. However, sometimes she opened her eyes. We did not believe she was seeing anything; comatose patients often open and close their eyes in response to the normal rhythms of sleeping and waking. Dick had an idea, though, that T just might be looking for something to see and nothing was there. He suspended a balloon over T's bed. Sure enough, T began to bat it back and forth with her hand. This was the first time she indicated any kind of response to her environment. Dick's mother said many times, "I'm so glad Dick noticed that she was tracking with her eyes and thought of suspending the balloon from the ceiling." I had no idea that this behavior was a precursor to her waking. As I have said, I had given up like everyone else. A few days after Dick had hung up the balloon, however, I was to receive a gift nine months in the making.

I walked into T's room and when she heard my voice she sat up in bed, opened her arms, and said "Mom." I was ecstatic. I made enough commotion that the nurses came running and suddenly we had a room full of doctors and staff members. They all came to see her and to share in our joy at her awakening. My T: Success Story.

T seemed in her element as they asked her question after question. Although she couldn't speak, she nodded for "yes," and shook her head for "no." She shrugged her shoulders for either "I don't know," or "I don't care." She almost seemed like the girl I remembered: that competitive teen going off to gymnastics.

There was a very proud look on her face as she responded to their questions. It was an amazing change that took place in a short period of time and even the professionals did not understand the abrupt transition. She pointed to her mouth and I realized she meant she was hungry. I started listing some of her favorite foods. When I said Big Mac, she excitedly nodded her head. While Dick went out to get the burger, it occurred to me that T had not eaten solid food for the better part of a year. The staff said that the worst thing that could happen is she wouldn't keep it down. T ate about half the burger and had a very satisfied look on her face. She had no problem digesting it. I called Renee to tell her T was out of the coma. She said, "I have to see it to believe it," and she flew out. Renee was amazed and delighted when T recognized her.

Suddenly I thought the sky was the limit. I assume I was not thinking about a full recovery, but I was so full of happiness that I just wanted to hold the feeling close. The medical staff was also excited and optimistic. Within a couple of days, though, I realized that my expectations for a complete recovery were unrealistic. It quickly became apparent that T had severe limitations with vision, speech, memory, and walking. Despite these facts, and they were facts, from the time T awoke until about a year later, I had false hopes. I deluded myself into thinking everything would be normal again. This was not to be the case.

We hired a neuropsychologist in Syracuse to test T. He tried various testing techniques. Her vision was not good enough for standardized testing, and he had to modify his evaluations to account for her lack of speech. T got basic orientation questions right but then it was hard to know if she really understood how she should answer. Although the tests were adapted, it was still extremely difficult to build a validity scale to obtain an accurate scoring. The doctor could not come up with specific answers.

What we did find out was that T sustained the most injury in the frontal lobe of her brain. This is where the executive function of the brain occurs and involves many aspects of higher thinking. She also had injuries in the back of the brain where the speech center is located and that is why she couldn't talk. Her memory was severely impaired. Her cognitive ability was in the range of an eight to ten-year-old. To complicate matters, T was now legally blind. This means different things to different people. For T, it meant she can see outlines and shadows only. We could never determine the extent of her vision impairment because of the difficulty with communication. Another interesting change that took place with the accident was what happened to T's hair. Previously blonde and straight, her hair turned dark brown and curly after the accident. No one seems to know why this unusual change has occurred.

We wanted to be with her as much as we could and even though the insurance company would only fund two trips a month, we flew there almost every weekend so we could be with her. After so long without her, I couldn't get enough of our time together. Initially, T's rehabilitation focused on walking. She progressed from a wheelchair to a walker by the time she was discharged. There was some emphasis on speech, but it was ineffective. The scans showed the damage to the speech area of T's brain was too severe. T ended up making up her own sign language to communicate with us.

Nicky, another young girl about T's age, was in a wheel chair and was in a nearby room. They would get together and have wheel chair races in the hallway. Although the elevator was by the nursing station, they would slip by the station, get in the elevator, and ride to different places. One day the staff, much to their consternation, found Nicky and T outside sitting in the plaza. Danger aside, I found it delightful and refreshing to see T exerting some independence. I thought, "That's my girl."

I had classes four days a week, four hours a day. I realized that if I really wanted to accomplish my goal of getting a Ph.D., I would have to stop working at the hospital to make it happen. I felt ready to move on anyway. I had been there a number of years, and the job was not particularly challenging anymore, so I resigned. In addition, T was coming back to Michigan, and we were putting her in a rehab facility close to our home. I would need extra time to visit her during the week and to bring her home on weekends.

I think one of the benefits of my educational experience was that it required total concentration in order to succeed. Therefore, when I was chipping away at the Ph.D., I was completely engaged in the task of the moment. The Buddhist philosophy talks about "being in the moment," and I was forced to do exactly that. I found that my class work was as effective as meditation in that regard.

Going back to school also helped me rekindle my social life. I made some life-long friends who didn't treat me like I was too fragile to be with. My previous circle of friends had fallen away because I had not had the time or inclination to socialize and when I did, it was awkward for both them and me. Many of my old acquaintances just didn't know how to react to me. They either ignored me or pitied me. After T's accident, I had very few people with whom I could connect.

One of the friendships I did have was with Helen. I met Helen at the Virginia facility. Her son, Brett, had sustained a traumatic brain injury in an alcohol-related accident just two days before T was hurt. Brett was also comatose, and Helen and I spent many hours commiserating and confiding. She would say to me, "If only Brett were like T," and I would realize the severity of our children's conditions was relative. Although the situation was not optimal with T, Helen made me aware it could have been worse. Coincidentally, Helen and her son lived in Michigan and were only about twenty miles away from our home, so we could maintain our friendship. I could always be myself with Helen; I didn't have to put on a false face and pretend that things were all right. We were simpatico. Helen was also a good sounding board for my dissertation, and I could test out my thoughts and ideas on her.

Dealing with being a student, visiting T, and getting other things in my life done required a lot of discipline, but it also gave me a perspective that empowered me. I remember one class on group therapy and no one seemed to be communicating. It hit me how hard T struggled to make her simplest thoughts known, and this group of intelligent, unimpaired people had all the ability and none of the desire to connect. They weren't even trying to find a common ground. I lost my cool and said, "I just returned from visiting a child who would give anything to be able to talk. You guys have all your faculties, and you still can't communicate; all you're doing is creating tension." They were completely silent, which was certainly better than speaking and saying nothing at all.

Completing the dissertation was a huge undertaking for graduation. I had conceptualized my research question, "What is the mother's experience of her child's traumatic brain injury?" but discarded the topic as being too sensitive. Then, a year later, I realized that no other research question had as much impact on me. This led me to wonder about how and whether other mothers came to terms with traumatic brain injury in their children.

As I began researching the topic, I became even more committed to my investigation of the phenomenon of being a mother of a traumatically brain injured child. I became aware of how little information professionals had on these mothers; mothers like me. In the end, I hoped my dissertation would help professionals understand what a mother goes through when her child has a brain injury and at the same time offer support to the family as a whole.

In addition to writing about my own experience, I met with and interviewed other mothers of brain-injured children. I began these interviews by explaining what a long journey it has been for me and sharing my hope that my research would help them and their families. I also gave assurance that I intended to help professionals better understand the needs of the family. These interviews were free-flowing, and I asked as few questions as possible to allow my subjects to have the interview focus on them.

What I found was that there were few striking differences between what each of the mothers experienced and felt. They voiced a large variety of specific concerns and issues, which I sorted and resorted and finally decided that most could be classified into four different categories:

1. Emotional issues and the grieving processes

2. Time issues seem insurmountable and greatly contribute to stress experienced by the family, particularly the mother, including managing time and balancing responsibilities as well as caring for a child who will not become a self-sufficient adult making the need for care seem like it will go on forever

3. Spiritual understanding: why has this happened?

4. Availability and depth of professional areas and support systems

The detailed findings in my dissertation are included in Part Two, Chapter 1.

CHAPTER 7:
GETTING ON WITH LIFE

After a couple of years, the medical staff at Arbordale in New York suggested T be closer to home, so we decided to transfer her back to Michigan. When T learned she was returning, she naturally thought she was coming to live with us again, which was what I wanted, too. Unfortunately, Dick and I were not of the same mind when it came to T's living arrangements.

Although we had undertaken the construction of a new, "T-Friendly" home, Dick was resistant to the idea of T moving in full-time. His idea was to house T in a rehabilitation facility and have her visit with us on weekends. I believe that Dick simply felt overwhelmed by T's condition; it was too much to handle. For my part, the idea that my child, my daughter, would be denied a home with me because she required care seemed abhorrent and wrong. I was her mother. She belonged with me. However, I had the sense that I could handle having T living elsewhere better than Dick could handle T living at home. In addition, it was hard for me to separate what I wanted from what might ultimately be good for T. I agreed to move her into a local pediatric group home, which was near our new house in Michigan.

Despite T's continuing desire to move home, we moved her from the pediatric group home to New Possibilities Rehabilitation when she turned eighteen. New Possibilities is one of the pioneers in brain injury care in Michigan. I would regularly drop in to visit her and check on things. I suspect the staff hated to see me "pop" in because I usually complained about something I thought they could do better. I had certainly changed from my soft-spoken, go-with-the-flow self. I may have had unrealistic goals as well since I believed only a mom knew what was best for her child.

Now that T was close to home, I would visit her during the week, and she came home most weekends. She loved being with us, and it was heartbreaking to return her to the group home on Sundays. Each weekend she visited, T thought she had come to live with us for good. I would die inside at her disappointment and sadness when I would remind her that she needed to leave because every time the hurt was fresh to T. Her memory and impaired executive function made it impossible for her to understand. Dick had managed to shield himself from guilt, or at least he seemed less affected when we dropped her off.

While she was at New Possibilities, T enrolled in a Special Needs high school program through the public school system where we resided. Since there was no teaching category for brain injury, they placed T with children with a variety of developmental and physical problems. They classified them as POOH (Physical Or Other Handicaps) but the program was really a dumping ground, and T was mixed in with all kinds of kids with all kinds of issues.

The high school situation wasn't optimal, but I think some of the social aspects were good. However, T was not happy and didn't want to go to school. She fought getting up and getting dressed. I wasn't actually sure why I kept insisting she attend, except that perhaps I knew there wasn't anything else that would fill her day. There were about ten children in her class. I started a note system with the teacher so that I could monitor what T did every day. The teacher responded in the notes with "Tania okay." The system was far from comprehensive but at least I felt somewhat involved. After four years, T got a diploma and went to the prom with a boy named Jay. Jay was one of her classmates who also had a brain injury and was deaf.

With some help from Patty, her musical therapist at New Possibilities, T composed this poem several years after she was back in Michigan:

> Sometimes I'm sad
> Cause I got hit in the head
> My head's gone so far
> I want to punch, slam and
> Punch
> Down below the floor
> Almost together
> Then apart
> Slam Slam

With T in New Possibilities in Michigan and after I spent four years in school, I eagerly looked forward to the end of classes. I wanted to complete my Ph.D. and move on with my new career. It was an exciting time, and I felt that all my hard work and study would pay off. At the same time, I knew I was facing another change, and the unknown was anxiety provoking in itself.

One of the requirements for graduation was to do an internship. I felt that doing an internship would be a good way to merge into the professional world. The Center assigned me to work at a substance abuse clinic. While substance abuse didn't particularly interest me, I thought it would be a good learning experience.

One of my clients had just been released from a drug rehabilitation program. At our first meeting, I suspected he was intelligent and based on his dress and vocabulary, I thought perhaps he was an executive. He was clean-shaven, and his light brown hair was styled in a short cut. He wore a well-coordinated LL Bean shirt and slacks. It was evident he cared about his appearance. His wife was in counseling about his drug problems and rehabilitation through another therapist in town. The therapist was educating her about how to help her husband. The wife was having difficulty actually perceiving the severity and seriousness of the situation. My client suggested that the four of us get together and discuss the situation as a group. We met and after some initial discussion, it was apparent that the wife didn't grasp the importance of the circumstances and her role in her husband's recovery. I asked her a pointed question, and suddenly the floodgates broke and she cried for about ten minutes. I can't exactly remember what I asked her, but it got to the crux of what was blocking her view of her husband's condition.

I finished that internship, graduated, and started planning my next step. I sent resumes to local clinics and remembered the practice that had treated my client's wife and sent a resume there, too. The therapist, Carolyn, immediately responded and asked me to meet with her. She said she was impressed with the way I had gotten through to the wife in our group session and this made her feel very positive about my skills. She explained her practice had grown too big for her to continue handling it alone, and she was thinking about referring some of her clients out. She invited me to share an office with her and take over some of her clients.

It was the perfect situation for me and we worked as a complimentary team. Carolyn didn't want to work evenings or Saturdays, so in the twenty hours I scheduled clients, I did mostly Saturdays and evenings. Her office suite consisted of two offices and a waiting area, but she had previously leased the second office to another therapist. For the first two years, we shared her office then the other therapist left, and I moved into the second office. I now work about thirty-two hours a week seeing clients and doing paperwork, and my hours span the week. It has been ideal for me and today, after twelve years, I am still working with her.

I also taught courses at a local college, the University of Detroit. I knew a therapist who was on staff, and she needed an adjunct professor to assist with teaching some of the classes. I taught introductory psychology to freshmen and sophomores. Since it was an elective course, all the students who were there chose to be there and were quite enthusiastic. I designed the classes to have student participation and interchange. The students always eagerly came through with interesting case studies since many of them had been teaching and had their own first-hand experiences to share. After about three years, I had to give up teaching when my practice got so big it didn't leave time for this activity.

CHAPTER 8:
ANOTHER CRISIS

My private practice was progressing nicely and although I still wasn't happy about T living at New Possibilities, I managed to live with the situation because I was able to drop in regularly and monitor T's care. Then Dick died suddenly of a heart attack in the spring of 1993. Although he had had by-pass surgery two years prior to this, a routine stress test the day before he died showed no problems. It was a total shock.

It was St. Patrick's Day, and we had gone out for corned beef and cabbage. We came home, and I noticed we needed a few groceries so I went to the store. I was gone less than an hour and when I returned, I called to Dick and got no response. I went upstairs and found him in front of the TV with his eyes open in a blank stare. I knew it was too late because he did not respond and although his eyes were open, they were staring off in space.

I ran downstairs and called 911. I called my daughter Renee and she said she and her husband Ali would be right over. Then I called my friend Judy who had a nearby farm, and she and her husband Bill came. They arrived when the paramedics did. I directed the paramedics upstairs. I still had my jacket on, and Bill asked if I wanted to take it off. I was numb and didn't want to take it off or sit down, as if not doing it offered some protection against the reality of the situation. After a while, one of the paramedics came down the stairs and said, "I'm sorry." I could not accept that he meant Dick had died. "No, do something!" I cried. He went back upstairs for a few minutes, then came back down and just said, "I'm sorry." I knew it was over. Renee's response was, "This is not happening."

Bill asked what I wanted to do about the funeral and said he had a friend who had a funeral home. He called his friend and took care of the preliminary arrangements. By then it was the early hours of the morning, so Judy and Bill went home, and Renee and her husband stayed with me. No one got any sleep. In the morning, Ali went out and brought donuts back for us. Then I called my friend Lynn, who was one of my classmates, and told her what had happened. She came over and went to the funeral home with me to select a casket and finalize the arrangements. The funeral director talked to us, but I cried the whole time and was thankful that Lynn was with me. She kept her arm around me and whispered things like "keep breathing" or "take a deep breath." Those simple words helped me tremendously. It was amazing how something as straightforward as breathing could be so helpful in a time of crisis.

Renee and I called people to tell them about the funeral. Renee asked if I could think of anyone else we should invite. "Yes, there was a minister at University Hospital who helped us when T was first injured," I said. "Do you remember her?" "Oh yes, Julie!" Renee responded. She called University Hospital and was able to reach her. Julie came to the funeral, and once again was a big comfort to us.

After the phone calls, Renee and I went to New Possibilities to tell T. Although the staff thought she would not understand what happened, I was sure she would grasp the severity of the situation, so I was apprehensive about telling her. She had a headache and was in the living room. She did have frequent headaches, and I do not know if this was a direct correlation to the accident or not. I said to her, "I'm sorry you have a headache because I have something to tell you that could make it worse. Your father has passed away." T screamed a sound that I have never heard from her. I just held her in my arms for a long time. When T had her accident, I thought, "Nothing could be worse than this." Nothing had been; not even cancer. Losing Dick; however, was worse than all of it. I cried all through the visitation and all through the funeral. One of the aides from New Possibilities came to the funeral with T and watched over her throughout this difficult time.

My clients were very understanding and accommodating. One of my clients had an appointment for the week after Dick died. When I told him I would keep our appointment, he asked me if I really felt I would be up to working. I thought if I could do something, it had to help the way I feel, and I did feel better. Fortunately, I had no crisis clients who needed immediate attention, so I was able to be flexible with my schedule.

Within a few weeks, T began withdrawing and I thought it best to have her see her psychologist, Dr. Reeves. He was a big comfort for T and helped her work through her fear that if she could lose her father, she could also lose her mother. Dr. Reeves took a special interest in T. He had a terrific sense of humor and could usually make her laugh. Dr. Reeves had mentioned that head injury victims often feel isolated and lonely. In fact, he said that loneliness is the primary problem with head injury victims. The professional literature supports this as well. At the 1991 Michigan Head Injury Conference I attended, it was emphasized that people can deal with memory problems, cognitive and physical problems, but the psycho-social aspects are the most devastating. These patients often feel so alone. Emphasis should be placed on three factors: work, leisure time, and close relationships. A relationship with another person is important so that the person with the head injury feels loved. Fortunately, or unfortunately, the loving often must come from the mother. T has developed a rapport with her psychologist over the years, and he has been invaluable when T goes into a depression. Although it is hard to know what is going on in her head, I believe she can become depressed when she realizes all she used to be able to do and how limited she now finds herself.

Strangely, over the years with the challenges I faced, I never felt the need for a psychologist until Dick died. His death ended a thirty-year marriage and thirty-seven-year relationship. I had to pick up the pieces without the one person who had always helped me do so. Renee was trying to establish her own life. She had finished law school and recently gotten married. She had her own career and life and did not need to take care of me. Dick had been such a big part of my life and despite any bumps in our marriage, he had always been there for me. I came from a very dysfunctional home. I met Dick when I was fifteen. In many ways, I felt as though he rescued me. He was always supportive of anything I ever wanted to do. We were a real twosome, and we always made decisions together. I didn't know what to do without him. Most of our friends were couples and although I kept in contact, I felt like a third wheel when I saw them. By the end of the summer, I realized I had fallen into a depression. I needed to do something about it because I needed to care for T. Fortunately, I found a gentle but forthright psychologist and she helped me slowly climb out of the hole. It really helped when she recommended medical support with a combination sedative and antidepressant. I felt better within a few months. At this point, T had been at New Possibilities for four years. All during that time, I had wanted to have T living with us at home, but Dick did not see how we could manage. Without Dick's feelings to consider, I decided to bring T home some time in the near future.

Chapter 9:
Tania comes home

I continued living in the house Dick and I built for a year after he died. I loved our house and the design among the trees but without Dick, it felt terribly isolated and remote. I couldn't see the neighbor's house and that added to the feeling of seclusion. Suddenly the whole wooded area had grown slightly menacing. I also wanted to be closer to Renee, so I began considering selling the house. Renee gave me the number of a friend who was a realtor. She suggested the realtor might be able to help me make a decision about what to do. The realtor came over, and we talked. I told her I wasn't really sure I wanted to sell the house. She suggested we list it to see what kind of traffic it got. We had an open house over the weekend and the first couple that saw it made an offer.

There was no decision to make about moving because the house was sold. After some looking, I found a house in Livonia, a near-by city, that I thought would work. It was closer to Renee and her family. I liked the house design, and the fact that it had a finished basement with a kitchen and living room closed the deal for me. The basement space had potential for a bedroom and the addition of a bathroom. Since I was contemplating moving T home with me, the basement area would be perfect for a live-in caregiver. I moved in, got settled, and decided to bring T home. She was ecstatic about coming home but also apprehensive and doubtful. I couldn't blame her because on so many occasions she thought she was coming home to live only to find out she was just visiting.

Bringing T home had its own set of problems and the initial adjustment was not always easy. I had to remodel the home to make it handicapped accessible and find caregivers. The insurance company was very accommodating about remodeling the house. They hired contractors to build ramps, place handrails on the tub, and construct a bathroom in the basement for the live-in helper I hoped to find. I was teaching two psychology college classes and running a part-time psychotherapy practice focusing on family therapy. For me, the main problem was finding how to schedule a life of my own while having T with me.

Trying to find people to help me with T until I found live-in help was stressful in itself. When I did find someone, there were problems with punctuality as well as knowledge and skills. This made work commitments almost impossible for me. Although I was not as worried about T as when she was at New Possibilities, I found myself taking my "mom thing" a bit farther than I needed, because I felt no one seemed to be better for T than I was. It seemed to me the other caregivers could not do her hair, nails, and clothes as well as I did.

Finally, after the frustration of trying to schedule various caregivers, I hired a live-in helper from Romania. Renee is an immigration attorney and found Vana for me. The positive part of the arrangement was that she was always there so I did not have to worry about my work schedule or other activities. The negative aspect was that it never completely felt like my home anymore, and I began to wonder whose home it was. I was not used to having live-in help. I treated her more like a guest than an employee. When I came home from work exhausted, I felt I had to chat. Indeed, her life was a lonely one so she was often bitter. Vana's English was not good. She did not drive and was often limited to the house with T. This was not an easy situation, especially given her personality. Romania is a third world country and living conditions are very poor. She told me that there was no room for abnormal children, so someone like T would have been completely forgotten in Romania. Vana was dour and humorless, and there was some relief when, after two years, Vana decided to return to Romania. After she left, I tried using several staffing agencies to provide caregivers and found varying results. Again the problem was both the quality of the workers as well as whether or not they would actually show up when scheduled.

One time when a suicidal client called, I needed to see her immediately and the caregiver had not shown up. Out of desperation, I took T with me and thought that I could leave her in the waiting room with some projects we had brought. Although I closed the waiting room door, T took to wandering the halls. Unfortunately, there was an unsympathetic therapist down the hall, who did not appreciate T's wanderings. While I understand he was working on his notes, a little more empathy would have been helpful.

Finally, I hired Brenda, a woman from the agency who was especially good with T. The whole situation improved. Brenda worked with T on Tuesdays, when I worked late, and Saturdays. Brenda also went to Florida and to a family reunion in Illinois to help with T. She felt like part of the family and is still with us today.

For a while, T and I continued living comfortably in the Livonia house. Brenda and various caregivers continued to help. My practice was building and meditation, journaling, and yoga were my key stress relievers. Then in 2002, the most unexpected thing happened to me: I fell in love. Although it had been several years since Dick's death, I never much thought of having a relationship with a man again. I was extremely busy keeping up with T and my clinical practice and didn't have time to have a relationship. Even if I were interested, I had no idea about how a middle-aged woman goes about meeting single, middle-aged men. Moreover, I had met Dick when I was fifteen-years-old and had never really dated anyone else. That was more than forty years ago. The whole thing was out of my league.

Nonetheless, kind of on a whim, a friend and I placed a listing on an Internet site. I was not very serious about the whole thing; it was my friend who was really pushing it. I chose a photo taken while I was making a ceramic tile, a new hobby I had discovered while camping on a weekend retreat. I didn't know I was being photographed, and my hair was in my eyes and my glasses were half off. That's how uninterested I was in meeting anyone.

As it happened, the ad turned out to be something that changed my life. A man named Chuck, who lived about thirty miles from me, read my ad. He saw it when he was visiting his only daughter, Liberty, in San Diego. He showed her several listings, and she pointed to my photo and said, "This is the one." Our love of cats was a common interest. He called me and when he returned to Michigan, we met for coffee. We talked for hours, but it seemed like minutes. His wife had died twenty years before and he had been single ever since. When we said good-bye that evening he said he would call, and I felt like a teenager waiting for the phone to ring. We started dating. The whole thing was so new and exciting for me. He later told me that he was taken with me the first time he looked into my eyes. Being with Chuck was extremely romantic.

Later that year, my father passed away and left his house to me. It was the house of my childhood in Birmingham, Michigan, in an old, quiet neighborhood with big, mature trees. You could see all the houses on the street, and each exhibited a character all its own. The house felt like home, and I thought T and I should live there. With Chuck's help, we moved from our Livonia home to Birmingham.

Chuck and I dated for a year and then got engaged to be married. We both had traditional, big weddings before and this time wanted a destination wedding. Six months later, we were married on an isolated, romantic island in Hawaii. Our dream of being married at sunset on the beach in bare feet came true. We both felt like we had been given a second chance at love and happiness.

Chuck moved in with me and T. It is marvelous to see the way he has taken to T. When he leaves, he gives T a hug, and she blows him a kiss. He does very well with the three of us living together. I am happy with the way things are working out. My practice is going well. I met other psychologists at a conference recently, and we have started meeting as a group. Because we are all in private practice, we find it valuable to share case work and information and to feel that we are growing professionally. Chuck and I are planning a trip to Germany in the fall. I believe we are coming together as a family.

With all this love around her, T has indicated she would like to have a relationship and have a special man in her life. She wants to be like her sister Renee and me. Rings symbolize love to her and are very important in her life. She has a large collection of rings and frequently points to her ring finger. When Chuck and I got married, T said, "What about me?" We tried to set up a dinner with Tim, a young man her occupational therapist knew, but it didn't work out. Once, when T and Brenda were in the mall, an attractive young man passed by and T turned to watch him. Although she is legally blind, there are some things that do not get by her. Brenda said, "Yes T, he is good-looking," and T became quite excited. She is interested, and we still have not ruled out a relationship for T. My yoga teacher likes to remind me that it has happened before.

CHAPTER 10:
TANIA'S RECOVERY

I was asked many times throughout T's recovery what my goals were for her. In the first few months following the accident, while she was in a coma, I only wished she could enjoy a Big Mac again, which she did. Aside from that, I always replied that I wanted there to be some quality of life for her. Now the quality of life I was hoping for is evident when she walks outside on a spring day and turns her face to the warm sun. It is also clear that quality is there when T leaves the house for the myriad of outings that now fill her life.

Today, I schedule as many activities as I can find that she enjoys. In addition to Brenda, I have found three young recreational therapists who take her on outings and their enthusiasm and energy is contagious. T loves going places with them and is delighted when the events going on around her are lively and full of energy. It is interesting that for some brain-injured people too much stimulation makes them very uncomfortable, but T thrives on it. The recreational therapists take T swimming and to movies and dances. They take her for pedicures and other activities that they think T will enjoy.

One of her favorite outings is shopping for "cool things": rings, jewelry, and anything pink. It's interesting that pink is her favorite color, since testing has shown that she cannot discriminate among colors. However, I suspect her intrigue with pink has more to do with the young caregivers who take her shopping and tell her that pink is "totally awesome." She also has a class in adaptive martial arts, which helps with her balance. We have a music teacher who comes into the home once a week. I am grateful that I have the means to provide all of this for her. I know others in my situation may not be as blessed, and all of these activities come at a cost, but love is always free. T started a scrapbook with pictures they take of all these activities. T has done all the cutting and pasting for this book, and it is truly beautiful. It is called "T's Memories." Her recreational therapists work with her on it and seem to be the key for her becoming more integrated. I only wish I had started with them earlier.

T visits New Possibilities two afternoons a week and over the years the services and outings have improved dramatically. Now she goes there for arts and crafts, and the staff is very interested in working with her. In addition, T has a job and works three days a week sorting parts. The business was started by a family with a head-injured member. Now they are willing to do special things to help others, like giving T a job. Her insurance company is also supportive of her emotional development, and they supplement part of her paycheck. It gives T a feeling of pride when she goes to work.

There is also an extremely special family near us that we met quite by accident. We were having lunch at a nearby restaurant. Our waitress was taken by T. She mentioned that she has a sister with Down's syndrome. Her mother also helps other special needs children so that parents can have some respite. She gave us the phone number, and we made an appointment to find out more. We arrived to find a wonderful farmhouse complete with horses. The whole family is involved. T spends at least one weekend a month with these special people. We are grateful to have found so many "angels" to spend time with T.

T is in a special needs church group and when I recently picked her up, the teacher had tears in her eyes. Someone asked a question, and T raised her hand to respond. She was able to sign the correct answer. This is something she had not done before. Then she lifted her hands in a prayer position looking up. This is what brought tears to the teacher. The expression on T's face was so pure it was almost beyond words. We learn unconditional love and being humble as part of our experience with T.

Brain injury is indeed a continuum. Progress is slow but changes continue to occur with T. Although it may not sound impressive, T can now use a straw which she could not coordinate before. In the last few months, people have asked what is different about T. This is because she looks so happy and content. She has so much more motor stability. When she gets up from sitting, she makes sure she is balanced and walks bringing the left leg out to coordinate with the right leg. Before she would just bring her right leg out and this put a great deal of pressure on her right side. I believe this improvement is because we sought some alternative therapies for her.

We have seen improvements with T in the past twenty-two years, but she still struggles with many issues. Loss of speech is the cruelest part of T's brain injury, since communication is our major link with the outside world. Through the years, T has had many speech therapists with varying degrees of success. She is still using a simplistic signing system, which probably does not express all that is inside her.

She has a voice system called DynaVox. She uses the Mini Mo model, which is a small portable communication device about the size of a computer keyboard. It allows T to use pre-programmed messages. It has a number of keys that play a pre-recorded message when depressed. Although T's memory interferes with her using it to its fullest potential, the keys have different textures to serve as a reminder of the message that they programmed on that key. Initially T would have nothing to do with the DynaVox. She wanted to speak on her own or not at all. However, her latest therapist Kate is very innovative and makes it more adaptable and fun for her. T now enjoys using it, and they are taking it to stores and restaurants to practice communicating. On Valentine's Day, one of the keys was programmed to say "I love you." When T pressed the key for selected people in her rehab building, she got a chuckle and a hug from them. This is quite a change in her behavior because T previously shunned both the DynaVox and her interaction with peers. She seemingly could not see herself associated with people who were disabled and regularly ignored them.

For a while, books on tape were a diversion for T. She enjoyed stories like "Little House on the Prairie" and "Eragon", an action-packed story about a boy and his dragon and magical powers. She intently listened to the American Girl tapes and was enthralled with their rich history. Although she loves stories, I am afraid we have used books on tape like some people use television to entertain their children. Now the newness has worn off, and it is difficult to find books she enjoys. Because of her memory problem, I often replay her favorite books. Sometimes that works and other times it doesn't. She often goes to sleep during the tape. I think this is withdrawing, but it is hard to know what is actually going on in her head and exactly how much she understands.

While at New Possibilities, T wrote this poem with the help of Patty, her former music teacher. It shows the insight T possesses about her condition:

The Dance of Life

When I was a child
Not such a long time ago

I felt the dance of life
And then had to let it go

When it takes for you
Your glass is always empty

The thirst is always there
The glass is like my body

Doesn't anybody care?

I've lost the way I used to dance
And laugh and sing and try

And sometimes when I look in the mirror

I just have to ask why

Patty helped her write this poem by giving T suggestions of words to choose from, and T would indicate the word she wanted to use. This writing is so insightful into the inner T and reminds me of how little I can truly share her perspective. It is easy for people to forget that T understands complex thoughts because she has only about ten hand gestures with which to communicate. I think this is because of her deficient memory. Most often, she communicates by responding to choices others pose to her. Her word recognition is actually sophisticated. When I read to her and ask her if she understands what a word means, she says she does. When I check her accuracy, she is correct most of the time. T was short-changed by fate and sometimes I feel pain for her that seems limitless. Having T at home, where I know how she is doing, relieves some of the ache inside me. I know she is happy to be with her family, so at least I can give her that.

Recently, T has become more cognitive. Her increased awareness has also increased her level of anger. The other day she had a scowl on her face and said she didn't want to go any place because she was angry. She also went out with one of her caregivers and started making distracting noises. Her caregiver reminded her that it was inappropriate behavior to display in public. I suspect some of this has to do with the fact that she may be maturing from cognitive age of eight to ten years, and is moving toward her cognitive teens, with all the accompanying defiance of the age. Before T's accident, as a thirteen-year-old, she didn't exhibit any of the oppositional behaviors common to teenagers, and I fear she's making up for that now.

Because of her recent behavior, we have T back in therapy with her psychologist. We recognize that T has little or no control over her life. She recognizes this as well and is very angry about it. We are trying to find things she can be in control of. This is often difficult. When we offer T choices, she will say "no" to each one and simply want to go to sleep. I am trying to be less controlling. For example, her caregivers and I are always cuing her to put her head up and not to slouch because it throws her whole body out of alignment. If she is lying down and I want her to sit up, she physically resists me. I think she is doing this for a sense of control in her life. Now, I am trying to let her be.

T wants to be involved in conversations, but we are not sure of how much she really understands what we are saying. The other day, Chuck and I were talking and he said he couldn't remember the name of a senator we were discussing. T raised her hand to sign, "I know," but it was difficult with signing to communicate with her. I do not think she really knew the name but wanted to be involved in the conversation. Another time, I was talking with Renee and I couldn't remember if our appointment was Tuesday or Thursday. Again, T said, "I know," and I asked her what she thought. She said it was Tuesday, but when I checked, I found it was Thursday. I knew at the time that T could not have known about my appointment, but I didn't mind consulting her. It seemed important for T to feel involved.

One of T's favorite quotes is by Helen Keller: "The best and most beautiful things in the world cannot be seen or even touched; they must be felt with the heart." T is legally blind. There is no doubt that she sees with her heart. T's Sunday school teacher noticed T seeing with her heart when she held her hands in prayer and looked purely to Heaven. We have seen T's "heart-vision" after watching/listening to a movie together. When justice triumphed, T stood up and clapped with that look of purity on her face. Through intuition or some kind of energy perception, T knows when there is a positive presence around her. She knows how I am feeling almost before I do. If I am not upbeat and laughing, she will put her arms around me and massage my neck. Love attracts her and illuminates her. T finds humor in the smallest things and has a contagious laugh. She loves to laugh at the expense of others, but without malice or unkindness. T finds it funny when another person has a moment that makes him or her seem more human. For instance, one day I put her shoes on the wrong feet, and she just laughed and laughed about it.

T has always had a competitive personality and excelled at most sports. This motivation to achieve, I believe, has helped her progress throughout her rehabilitation. She still loves to win. Winning can be as simple as me saying, "You are right; I didn't figure that out quite as well as I should have." T wins when a choice or decision she made was the correct one. For instance, if she chooses the I-Max movie we will see and after the movie, we all agree it was a good movie, she gets a gleeful look on her face and chuckles with victory. Her laugh really is music to my ears. Because of her sight deficit, her hearing has become extremely acute. T was in another room when I whispered something to Chuck only to hear T chuckling in the other room because she heard what I said. There are no secrets from T.

Upon reflection, I am not sure we ever get used to this new child, no matter how long it has been. Ever since that April evening, the initial words of the neurosurgeon at the University of Michigan Hospitals keep coming back to haunt me. "If she wakes up, you will wish that she had died," she said. Well, T is awake and I don't want her to die. I often wonder if this is selfish. I cannot discern what she thinks and feels about her future. Can she even hope and plan?

My life was very comfortable before the accident. Daily activities took on a sameness that, in retrospect, was reassuring. A large part of today's drama is of course T. She works very hard in whatever challenge comes her way in the rehabilitation process. This is very much like the pre-accident T: ready to take on any new challenge. It is only lately that I catch a resigned look in her eye. In my heart, I am crying, "T, don't give up." However, I sense she is tired. It is as if she is saying, "I have tried so hard. I have done everything that people have asked me to do. I even asked for more shots and medicine thinking in my mind that they would make me well again and change me back."

When T awoke from the coma, I felt intense joy. She knew who I was and was in contact with our reality. This was followed by the bitter disappointment of looking at a sunset and seeing the pink hues and believing that T cannot enjoy this beauty. We cannot yet tell if she remembers or discerns color, never mind the understanding of beauty. Communication is the mainstay of mankind. T is now robbed of this basic right.

Still, as I write this, I am aware that T really needs to be in control. She has lost so much control over her life that she will react in a negative manner just for the feeling of getting it back. She can be very adamant about assuming control. She has developed a cough that she displays at will. We've had her checked medically for congestion and allergies, and T had a clean bill of health. A caregiver recently had T at the movies, and she must have been bored. She went into a coughing fit. The staff took her to the lobby to get her water. When the staff returned with the water, the coughing started again. Of course, the caregiver interpreted this as defiance. T has very few ways to gain control, and I think coughing is one way to get it. In addition to coughing at the movies that day, T soiled her pants in the car. This is something she never does and when they got home, the caregiver was angry and looked to me for consequences for T. The caregiver suggested no movies for a month. I knew that would not serve a purpose; T's memory index reaches seconds not weeks.

When these incidents occur, I might feel negative about them. However, it is sometimes easier to glean humor from the situation. This often occurs later. I find if I can relax and lighten up about the situation, it generally has a more positive outcome. For example, once T was having trouble sleeping. I was almost asleep when I heard her moving around. I found her sitting on the living room couch with her purse and her shoes on, apparently ready to go. She had no inkling about where she wanted to go. She used the sign of turning a wheel for driving. She also flapped her arms, which means she wants to fly on an airplane.

I understand that each brain injury case is different. However, for a child such as T, lack of control must be devastating. Pre-accident T was a very take-charge, directed type of kid. Now that control in her daily life is gone.

Between her laughter and her heart-felt presence, I do know that I have someone special and precious in my life. What would it be like if she were more like her able bodied peers? I can only speculate. Because she was only thirteen at the time of the accident, time is on our side. She is young enough to benefit from research and new techniques continually being discovered. I know in my heart that T will continue to evolve. I do not know what form that will take, but it will be my T. Is she really limited?

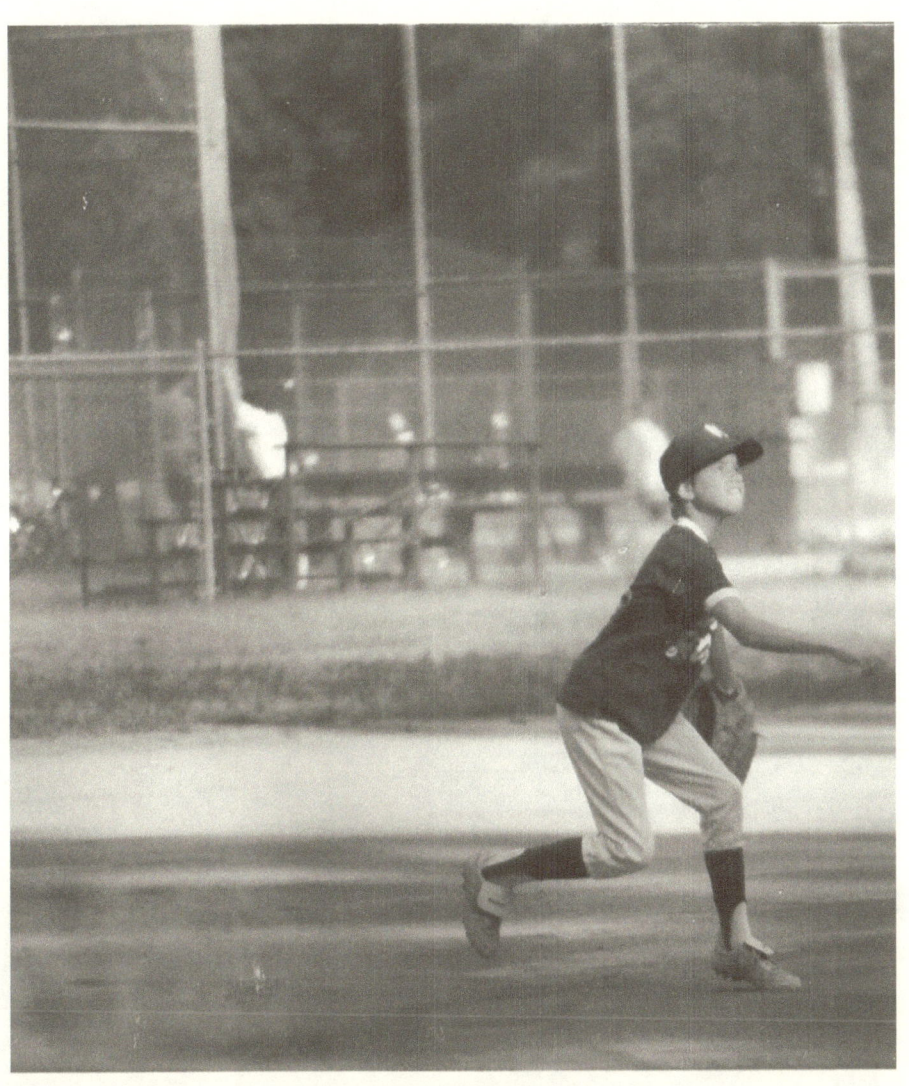

Before the accident, Tania played softball.

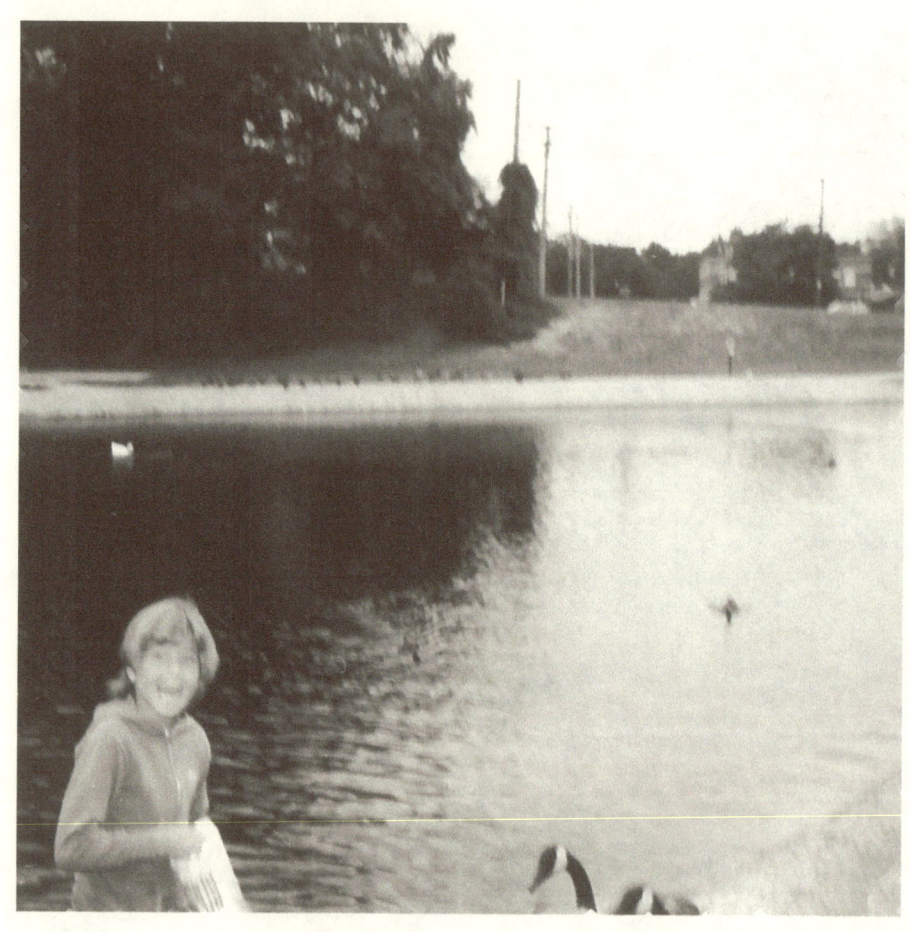

Tania loves animals and got a great thrill feeding them.

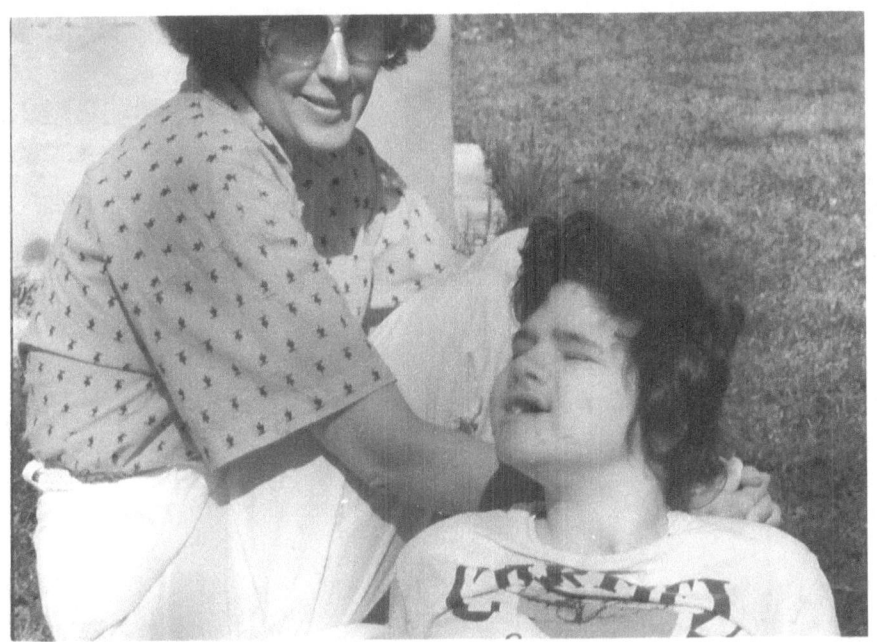

Tania with her mom soon after the accident. Tania enjoys the sun on her face.

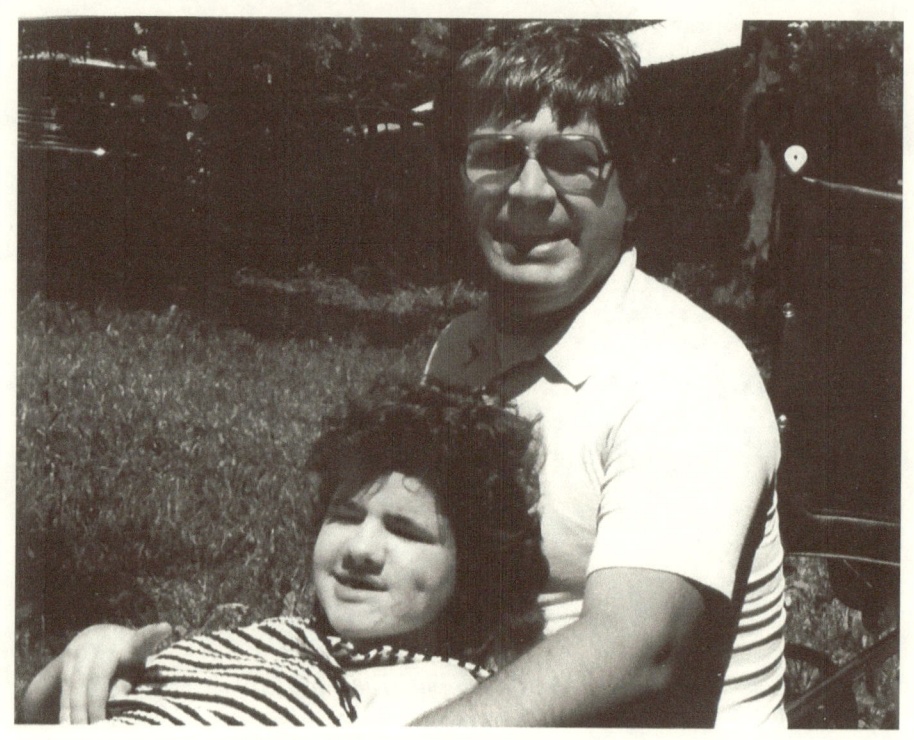

Tania with her dad soon after the accident.

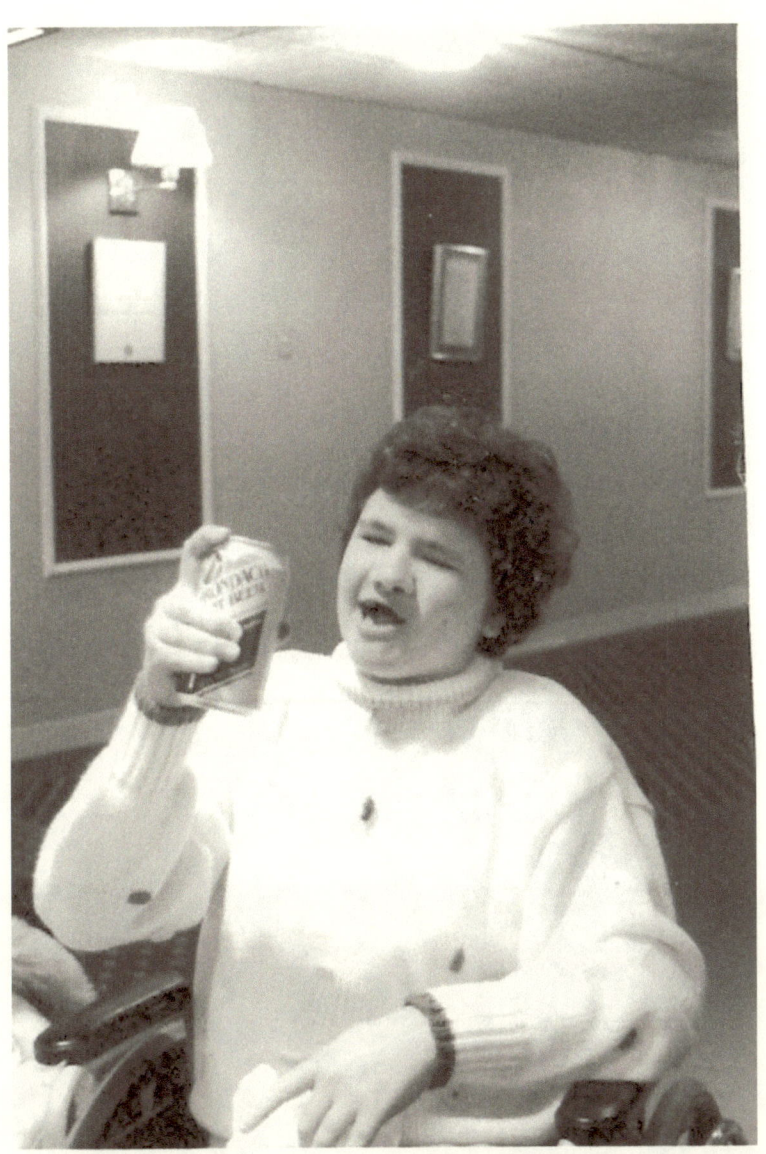

Tania drinking a soda in the hallway of the facility where she lived.

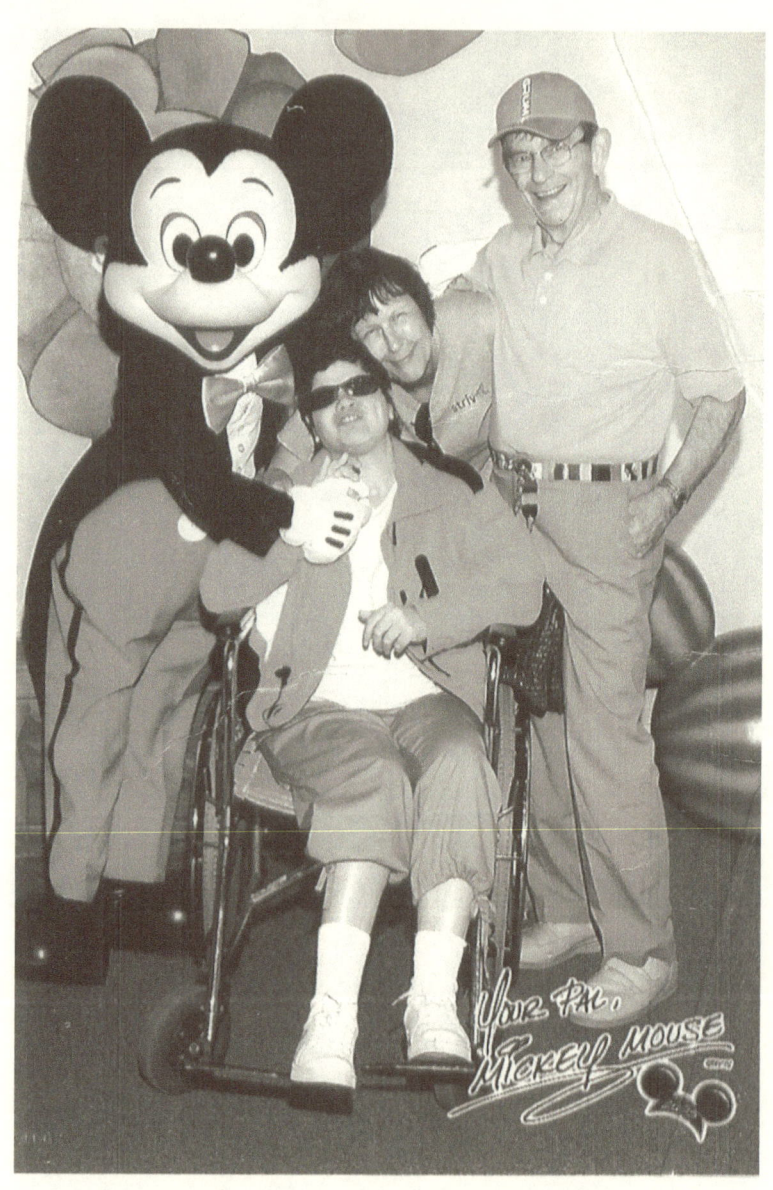

Tania at Disney World with her mom and step-father Chuck.

PART TWO:
WORDS OF WISDOM

Chapter 1:
Dissertation findings

I realized as I was writing this book that I have been fortunate in many respects regarding this most unfortunate of situations. I was lucky in the sense that I had many resources on which to draw support during T's hospitalization, rehabilitation, and subsequent and continuing care. The state of Michigan has no-fault insurance which means your car insurance automatically takes responsibility for your care if you are injured in an auto accident. They have a catastrophic account which provides funds for many of the things T requires. Also, my family had, and has, the means and the wherewithal to provide T with activities that enrich her life as much as possible. In many cases, perhaps in your own, resources are not affordable or available. I am aware that the financial burden placed upon families of children with traumatic brain injuries can feel daunting and insurmountable. Many others in my situation are not so fortunate and all these activities come at a cost, but love is always free.

In addition, I am writing from the perspective of hindsight and emotional distance that comes with the passing of time. I have the benefit of being over two decades down the road from T's initial accident and have gone through my own recovery as a result. I need to assure you that the narrative you have just read in no way can describe the pain and hopelessness that we felt, and that you may be feeling now.

It may help you to know that I could not have written this book without the passage of time to serve as a buffer between my intellect and my grief. Wherever you and your family may be in the process, I have been, and still am, somewhere along the same path. The story of T and our family is a work in progress, and I am sure that there will continue to be challenges ahead that I will have to learn to overcome. For now, I hope our story has helped you feel as if you are not alone and that the following chapters can give you some tools to make your life easier. When I began to research my dissertation question, "What is the mother's experience of her child's traumatic brain injury?" I believed my findings would either confirm or disprove many of the assumptions I had made about my own experience with T. It felt like the right decision and, as I reflected on the previous year, I realized how absorbed I had been in this topic. It was always foremost in my thoughts whether I was going to class, shopping for groceries, sitting by T's bedside, meditating, or journaling. My journal consisted entirely of reflections in the form of letters to T. I read everything I could find on brain injury and constantly wondered about what other mothers were experiencing. It then became clear to me that choosing this topic would not only help me gain some insight and understanding into my own experience but that the information could potentially help other families and professionals as well. So I decided to pursue that topic and set up my inquiry to involve the following three phases:

- *Immersion into my own experience.* I totally delved into processing my experience by journaling, mediating, and staying totally focused on the moment. I found the more I could do that on both an emotional and objective level, the clearer the situation became to me. I found that resistance to process caused part of the stress I experienced. I thought about what was going on in my life and what I needed to do about it at the time. It was with full awareness of what I was doing that I jumped into my dissertation project.

- *Examination of the literature.* I searched to find the information currently available about the mother's experience, and this exploration revealed that very little material existed. I did find some information about the stages the family goes through with an emphasis on denial, guilt, grief, and depression.

- *Exploration of the nature and meaning of the mother's experience.* I found mothers who agreed to interviews so I could obtain the essence of their experience and compare and contrast them. I briefly told them about my experience with T and explained that I wanted to hear about their experience. I tried not to ask them questions so that I did not lead them in any particular direction.

INTERVIEW SUMMARIES WITH MOTHERS OF CHILDREN WITH A TRAUMATIC BRAIN INJURY

The following are interview summaries of mothers with a traumatic brain injury and their experiences (names have been changed to protect privacy):

Pat

Pat said her son Marcus is unable to communicate and does not know who he is. It is imperative that someone else meets all of his needs. He is able to pick up finger food if it is in the right place but if it's placed six inches to the right, he would starve to death just looking at it. She had a profound sense of frustration over the lack of progress she sees with her son. Marcus was in an out-of-state rehabilitation facility for over a year because there was not an adequate facility in their state. This added to the stress and after a year, the family decided to bring him home. Pat said her other children virtually went to high school on their own because she was so preoccupied with Marcus. Her daughter never brought friends home because Marcus would make loud grunting noises and roll around on the floor and this embarrassed her. Pat's daughter has a lot of hatred toward her mother for ignoring her. Pat's other son never played sports because he was periodically filling in as caretaker for his brother. Pat said if she wanted to relax and read at night, she thought Marcus was sad to be alone. If she was going shopping, Marcus would go too. Pat tried to make sure he looked as cool as possible, dressed in the best clothes and shoes, just like with their other kids. Her marriage almost fell apart. Therapy helped them realize they needed to move Marcus out of the house. He left home for the summer, and they saw "how there was not much of him there." It was a slow process coming to that realization. In the fall, they panicked when they realized they couldn't bring themselves to take him back. "We could finally enjoy TV, have the house to ourselves, and go out for dinner," she said. Then she reflected that with all her hard work during the previous five years, she never made her son any better. "I have never met a parent who did not wish for a miracle to happen," Pat said. "We are all nuts and nothing is ever going to be good for us until he can be better." Pat remembered a doctor asking her three times how she was doing until she finally broke down. He got her into counseling, and her psychologist was very good at stress management. This was the first time Pat felt that a professional had helped her. Pat cries at weddings because Marcus will never get married, have kids, or go to college. However, it gives her some comfort that he does not appear to be unhappy. She is concerned about his future and does not know what the answer is. Although Pat was raised Catholic, religion has not helped her. She feels envious of those whom religion helps. "It gets them through a lot of pain," she says.

Dana

Dana's son Kevin remains unresponsive to the environment four years after his accident. Dana has finally gotten to the point of acceptance where she knows that her son is not going to change dramatically. She thinks that is a healthy place for her to be, especially when she reflects on parents she met who are still in denial. Dana believes denial can be very limiting. She admits she was in denial for a couple of years before she "reworked her life." Dana feels her son "basically died in the accident." She addresses the isolative grieving process for a person who still lives and finds it hard to describe. It is as if through this partial death "he is inside this new person." Dana is extremely pessimistic about the future and says it hurts beyond what she can say to imagine that the situation will never change. Thinking about the way Kevin exists is too immense for Dana, and she said thinking about it, "makes me wish he had died." She has an immense sense of being overwhelmed. Dana describes herself as walking around in a fog for four years. She believes the fog helped distance her from the pain of loss. She says, "The pain runs so deep that I cannot even see it. Nothing can fill it." The pain is so prominent in her life that she reflects on the situation as an ongoing nightmare. "I would not wish this on my worst enemy," she says. "It is that bad." Dana's relationships changed after Kevin's accident. She became involved with an alcoholic, which was a diversion for her. She did not have to face how bad Kevin was. "There was someone there to hold me," she said. She desperately needed comfort and could not think clearly about the source. Dana realizes a part of her died in the accident and that she will never get all of that part back. Fortunately, a psychologist helped Dana focus on herself so she stopped putting all her energy into what her son had lost. Her grieving became more intense, however, because she was grieving not only for her son, but for herself and what she had lost. She knows she needs to take care of herself and attempts to balance self-care with spending time with Kevin. One side of the scale is caring for herself; the other side is dealing with the guilt she feels when she does not see Kevin. Dana spent a great deal of time contemplating how a tragedy such as this could occur but has accepted that she will never figure it out. She is sustained by her belief in God; although she said it has been a real test of her faith.

Nancy

Nancy describes the essence of her experience by detailing her son Dean's day-by-day experiences. She said he retains very little information but occasionally remembers something that has some interest to him. Once, she told him she had purchased a Buick LaSabre. Later, when he asked what car she would be driving when she picked him up, she answered, "the Buick." Nancy was surprised when Dean then said, "Oh, the LaSabre." Nancy also describes Dean's physical actions, another facet of the essence of her experience. Dean has an oral sensitivity that manifests by his chewing almost anything, including paper. She sounded slightly detached as she described how his shirts would sometimes be in rags from Dean's chewing. Dean had a tremor in his right arm and would not write for two years. Now, Dean writes only when necessary. If handed a pencil, Dean cracks it in half and throws it. However, he will type on a keyboard and will use a Speak and Spell for hours. The Speak and Spell is something over which he has control, and he doesn't get bored because he doesn't remember what he has done on it. Nancy has divided feelings about several things. It took a long time for her to accept any credit for Dean's progress. The future concerns her, and she says, "I'm not going to be here all his life." Then she says she couldn't trust someone else to look after him. Nancy wants to know where he is all the time. She says that if she puts an addition on the house she would know where he is. Then she realizes that if he were home she "probably would not survive." She realizes that he would not reach any independence at home because it is difficult for her to watch his slow progress when completing tasks. Inevitably, Nancy takes over and performs the task for him. Nancy doesn't think there are answers. When she visits Dean, she grapples with fatigue and guilt. On the other hand, she goes for three weeks without seeing him because it is so exhausting. She says, "By the third week, it just kills me." She expresses aloneness and isolation. She cannot talk to other people because "the only person who could understand is someone with a head injured family member." Nancy asks "why" and tries to come to grips with her situation by seeing some good come from talking with and supporting other parents of head-injured children. Nancy reflects that this is "a terrible why."

Brenda

When Brenda arrived at the hospital, she explained she was not the legal guardian, her husband was. The staff member responded, "It is okay, you are the mother. Sign." She received a $120,000 judgment against her, and the state of Michigan demanded she pay up or surrender her driver's license, car registration, and her license plates. "For a long time I was in a really bad state," she said. She never sought to regain custody; she had Keith. The father never contributed unless he wanted to exercise some control. Brenda is now afraid of her son Keith. His radio became his security blanket and one night it was blasting at 2:00 AM. She went to the basement fuse box, pulled the fuse, and did not go back upstairs that night. Keith was banging on the door. The next morning she denied taking it out. "That's how intense it was," she said. Brenda now has a problem driving and when traffic is heavy, she gets off the freeway. This adds extra time to her travels. One day she was so edgy, she turned around, went back home, and asked her other son to drive her. Brenda remembers crying and crying. "Trauma, agony, and suffering; boy, does it hurt," she said. A part of the pain emerges when she sees Keith's friends having fun and says it just tears her apart. She sees the endless quality to her experience. "This will not go away; this nightmare will go on forever. Your whole life is to be a mother," she adds. She has become aware of how women are often nurturing others at their own expense. Initially she was against a group home. For the first time, Brenda learned that love is not a cure-all. Yet, Brenda searches for the bright side to what has happened and thinks a study group can use Keith to help other people understand. "A couple years ago, a person like this would not have survived," she said. "If Keith eventually has some quality of life that would be good, but I can't see any reason for 'them' surviving." It was not until several years after the accident that Brenda felt herself "mending." She searches for a quality of joy in her life but the cloud of despair caused by Keith's accident obscures the light of any joy for Brenda. She found counseling hard to accept at first, since she views herself as a strong person and "the mother who has weathered all the storms." She finally did accept counseling and found that it helped her cope.

Dolores

Dolores said her experience was "Horrendous, horrendous. I just cannot put it into words. It was such a hard road back; we all had to rebuild our lives." She recognized how much denial is involved in attempting to come to terms with her son Allen's accident. "You just want it to be a dream and wake up to find everything is all right," she said. In an effort to put her experience into words, Dolores wrote this poem:

A Mothers' Prayer

God, bestow your patience
Upon my soul today
My son lies in a coma
And all I do is pray

My bodily needs forgotten
My soul aches deep inside
Should you reveal some light
I surely will abide

The moments as he lies there
I suffer just the same
The only subtle difference
I answer to my name
Grant a ray of hope to me
Don't take his life today
For then I'll comfort others
Knowing what to say

Dolores remembers feeling despair, as if she were going through a long, black tunnel. For a long time, she could see no light at the end. It all seemed so hopeless that she could only see the blackness of despair. To cope, Dolores found solace in finding ways to help Allen. She is very angry at the state programs, which were not helpful. Professionals called her "overbearing" when she advocated finding services for her son. "Professionals just shut you out; I had to beg to get Allen into programs," she said. "These people rob you of your dignity." For Dolores, a big part of the pain is thinking about the brilliant future Allen might have had. "We had such high hopes," she said. "But it was not meant to be." This indicates a type of acceptance, not that it is all right, but that it just is. Dolores said when Allen returned to school, the personnel did not realize he had problems with his memory and learning new information. They gave him a full load of class work, which he was no more ready for "than the man in the moon," Dolores said. Allen quit school but returned later to take one course. The thing that helped Allen most was his friendship with the librarian at school, who was a very caring man. The librarian took an interest in Allen, and he would seek the librarian out when "things got to him." The librarian owned two bookstores, and Allen was a frequent customer. Because the librarian cared about him, Allen began to care about himself and feel worthwhile.

Debbie

Debbie's thirty-four-year old son Jon was injured six years ago while driving a motorcycle without a helmet in Seattle. "I flew out in a snowstorm and even though I am deathly afraid of flying, I never gave it a second thought," Debbie said. She only knew that Jon was seriously injured. "Although I am Catholic, I could not pray. I did not know what to pray for." When she arrived at the ER, Jon was in a coma and ready for surgery. The hospital staff told Debbie there was no hope; then she knew what to pray for. Jon was in surgery for almost eight hours. Debbie said initially she was in denial. She told the people from the head injury organizations to leave her alone; she had other things to do. She gave all the pamphlets pertaining to head injury back to them. She was listening to what the hospital staff said about what needed to be done for Jon to become functional. They started physical therapy practically as soon as he came out of surgery. Debbie stayed with Jon in Seattle for two and one-half months. Her husband came out for awhile but had to return to Michigan. Debbie knew she could not stay in Seattle forever, but she still wanted to oversee Jon's care. There was no insurance. Since the accident happened in Seattle, Seattle would have assumed the responsibility for his care, in a nursing home or other facility. Although Debbie is not exactly sure how it happened, hospital personnel contacted the state of Michigan and explained the situation, particularly the stress it was causing to have the family separated. Michigan agreed to assume responsibility for him. That is quite a liability because even if the person receives Medicaid, it is for a lifetime. Debbie was told to apply for Disabled Social Security for Jon and had heard horror stories about the process. However, the woman from Social Security was very helpful, and even invited Debbie to go out to dinner. Debbie feels it does no good to live her life on "ifs and maybes," but says she never looks at Jon without remembering the way he used to be, and it still hurts a lot. "I could not look at a photo album for years because it hurt so much to remember how he was." Jon's long-term memory is good, so he remembers, too. Debbie disagrees with people who say you should accept the new person and leave the old person behind. "Part of that person is gone forever, but he has not totally died," she said. "Part of that person is still here with feelings, likes, and dislikes. It's not fair to bury the person who was before. Then what do those pictures in my photo album mean? Those are memories of the way that person was." Professionals have shown Debbie a lot of kindness, but she feels they do not really understand head injury. "I find it very difficult to go to the conferences and listen at some of the workshops," she said. "They are trying to tell us something we know, and I don't think I'm alone in thinking when I leave that I come away with more unanswered questions. I know so much more; not because I am smart or a smart ass but because I live it. I think the people in rehabilitation facilities do not understand. They work an eight-hour shift and go away from it, and we do not. As mothers, it stays with us until we die." Debbie and her husband have seven children and Jon is a middle child. They are concerned about what will happen with Jon when they can no longer care for him because he is very dependent. His brothers and sisters told the parents not to worry, but that is neither what they want for Jon nor their other children. They want them to go on with their lives, and they want Jon to get on with his life. However, funding is an issue. "I think Jon could be made into a useful human being; he works on a computer quite well," Debbie said. "We have a tutor who works with him on software and makes assignments." Jon cleans his room and takes care of his own laundry, but it took over a year to teach him to make his bed. He is always making progress. It may be in very small increments. You have to be consistent. Don't think I did not get frustrated and screamed and hollered because I did." Debbie says she rarely has time for herself and feels stuck. She gets angry with Jon and then recalls that Jon does not remember. She feels the longer he is with them, the more dependent he will become and it is unfair to him. "I feel like when I have accepted the way things are, something kicks me in the behind, and it is all new and fresh," Debbie said. "That is the horrible thing about head injury; it never goes away."

INTERVIEW SUMMARY

I want to emphasize that I found inner strength and courage, not just in the mothers, but in their children as well. Yes, there is pain and struggle, but it is amazing how the human spirit, when put to the test, can survive and cope. I watch T struggle to walk and understand her new, limited world, and I am amazed at how the human spirit strives to grow in the bleakest of circumstances. T expresses her struggle in the following poem:

Now by Tania Burgess

Now the anger rushes
Through me
Like a tidal wave that destroys
My control is slipping away
What happened to all the joy?
The changes are many
The most important thing that
Remains the same
Is the love and support of my parents
But even through that love
I still feel the same

The process of interviewing these mothers contained a therapeutic element for me. The rich sharing we did created a bond between each of them and me. Truly, no mother who has not experienced losing part of her child to a traumatic brain injury can really understand what it is like.

In reflecting deeply on these interviews, I envisioned the quilt that my grandmother made. She had nine daughters. When the cotton dresses became too small for the youngest daughter, they became pieces, then blocks, of these quilts. Writing the synthesis was like sewing together the quilt. Each stanza was carefully drawn from one of my interviews; therefore, each stanza is one mother's attempt, including mine, to piece together her experience of partially losing her child. Together they make an integrated design. Each part taps into the inner rhythm of the experience and enhances the completed design.

Beyond Hurt by Mary Burgess

This endless nightmare
of looking for the missing pieces
to a puzzle that once was
    Tania

Dear Science: I offer you a prayer
    There is so little left of him
    Please put your time, energy and money
    into making him whole again

Why didn't you die?
What do you have to teach us?
Can our struggle give strength to others?

This isolative, secret
    Grieving process
    for one who still lives
    I know you know my touch
It is not enough

I hate you God
    She lies in a coma
    I have lost my love for you
    You, who were supposed to care for us
    There is silence

Deep in my heart
I would bring him home
    But, I wouldn't survive

You still feel, like and dislike
I can't bury the boy in the photos
It would not be fair to those pictures

I am stuck
   In an endless fog
Who will be there for you someday?

I see your friends
   having fun
It tears me apart
But I am mending

I thought the birds would sing
and I'd never enjoy them again
But I found my solace
   in helping you

SYNTHESIS OF INTERVIEWS

When I finished the interviews, I wrote every issue that we discussed on a 3 x 5 card. I sorted and re-sorted them hoping to come up with some common themes. I found I could divide each issue into one of the following four categories:

1. Emotional issues and the grieving processes

2. Time issues seem insurmountable and greatly contribute to stress experienced by the family, particularly the mother, including managing time and balancing responsibilities as well as caring for a child who will not become a self-sufficient adult making the need for care seem like it will go on forever

3. Spiritual understanding: why has this happened?

4. Availability and depth of professional areas and support systems

Emotional issues and the grieving process

Families struggle first with the hurt and pain. Most are in some state of denial, and there is the grief that they experience in losing a part of the person they love. One author, Sandy Souza, a mother from Texas with a child with a brain injury, wrote that brain injury is not like death because there is no resolution but a continuing state of limbo. With death, there is an end and subsequent action of continuing with life. In the case of caring for a person with a brain injury, the situation goes on forever and has to be addressed, in one stage or another, for a lifetime. The individual who suffered the brain injury remains partially present, as a constant reminder of the loss.

Another article by a researcher, Judith Mitiguys, stated that a child's brain injury shatters or severely alters dreams that parents have for their children. As Pat, one of the mothers I interviewed, said she cries at weddings because her son will never get married, have kids, or go to college. This is just one more way that a family grieves.

A mother might talk of a "hole in my heart that can never be filled," and pain that "runs so deep, I cannot even see it." They say they feel devastated, lost, empty, depressed, hatred, anger, and guilt. They feel stuck, in a fog; they are "going through a long black tunnel and that it feels like a burden." Chapter 2 has more information on grief and denial.

Time issues seem insurmountable and greatly contribute to stress

Time issues seem insurmountable and greatly contribute to stress experienced by the family, particularly the mother, including managing time and balancing responsibilities as well as caring for a child who will not become a self-sufficient adult making the need for care seem like it will go on forever. The mother of a child with a traumatic brain injury feels heavily burdened with responsibility. Time management is difficult and at times it is impossible to finish all that needs to be done. She wants to make sure she is doing as much as possible for her child but at the same time, she realizes the importance of taking care of her own needs. However, many mothers are not able to balance responsibilities and do not find the time to get relief in any way. Mothers said that the accident seems to have changed the way they think about time. Sometimes if feels like fifty years, and sometimes it feels like yesterday since the brain injury occurred. Thinking a year ahead is too immense when they realize the nightmare they are experiencing will stay with them until they die. Many describe the situation as an ongoing nightmare that will not change dramatically and makes them feel pessimistic about the future. Along with that they wonder what will happen to the children when they are no longer able to care for them. The management and perceived endlessness of time contribute greatly to the overwhelming stress families, especially mothers, experience. Because this issue is so important, I have devoted chapters 4, 5, and 6 to stress.

Spiritual understanding: why has this happened?

According to the mothers, families search for greater meaning from the accident and ask why this tragedy has happened to them. There are also spiritual aspects associated with this, and some people have found religion to be a useful coping mechanism. The attempt to discern why this terrible thing has happened is part of each mother's experience. No one seems to have found any good answers.

Availability and depth of professional areas and support systems

Families found that often the medical community really didn't understand what they were experiencing with a family member with a brain injury. As a result, professionals were often of minimal assistance in providing needed help or resources. Mothers did occasionally find comfort in counseling.

Professionals play a role in the mother's life from the first day of her child's accident and continue to do so for as long as the mother and child live. It is important that professionals stay attuned to new knowledge in their field, as it relates to head injury. All too often, mothers have encountered professionals who seem to know too little about brain injury. I say this based on my own experience and the discussions, comments, and questions from the mothers themselves. Mothers also commented that when they went to professional conferences concerning head injuries, they often knew more than the speakers who were presenting information. The professional community still has not adequately dealt with these issues. Many of the issues cited here will be addressed in subsequent chapters.

CHAPTER 2:
WHAT I HAVE COME
TO REALIZE

The following are the things I have come to realize and understand about living with a brain injury. Subsequent chapters in Part Two elaborate or offer suggestions on family dynamics, stress, and coping.

REHABILITATION IS LIFE LONG

I think the most important thing for people to understand when dealing with a brain injury in their family is that recovery is a life-long process. Improvements do not occur as quickly as we would like but continue to occur throughout the patient's life. Rehabilitation is a relearning process. Ideally, rehabilitation trains other brain neurons to take the place of those that have died, and it can take years for function to return. All of the mothers I interviewed commented on how progress is gradual and comes in small increments. The question of how much a person is expected to recover from a severe brain injury was never answered for me. I now understand that recovery depends on several factors, the most important points being the areas of the brain that were injured and the duration of the coma.

Initially, I had a difficult time with the rehabilitation process. Looking around the therapy room at the other patients made me wonder what T was doing there. I was still in denial and not willing to accept that she belonged with these people. It hit me hardest that T was no longer the child I had known when I sent her to an art camp. When I picked her up, I found her slumped over in her chair, unaware of her surroundings. The old T would have been running around showing others what they were supposed to be doing.

I have found part of the life-long rehabilitation process is to keep looking for new techniques and alternatives that may be helpful. I constantly try new things or revisit things we previously tried, but present them in a different way or with a different person. For example, T had tendon-release surgery to ease the spasticity in her ankle that was a result of the brain injury. It was only partially successful, and she still needed to swing her right side out to walk. The movement created enormous muscle tension as well as a wobbly gait. Recently, we started using massage therapy, polarity, and Reiki healing. This has made a big difference in the way she walks as well as alleviating some of her discomfort.

In addition, the patient needs to learn other adaptive skills, physical as well as emotional. Today, many years later, I see shifts in increased adaptations in T. For instance, she is now using the DynaVox Mini-Mo voice machine, which she previously ignored. I believe she is using it now because a new teacher found a way to make it appealing to her.

EMOTIONAL ISSUES FOR THE PATIENT ARE IMPORTANT

It is important to address the isolation and loneliness people with a brain injury often experience. They need to feel emotionally supported, as well as have a sense of self-worth and dignity. T isolated herself from other people with brain injuries and for many years, she shunned and ignored them because she felt she did not belong with them. Recently, however, she has become much more interactive with her peers. I have no idea why her attitude changed, but I am encouraged by this because I know it eases her isolation and loneliness. As T's psychologist has pointed out, emphasis should be on work, leisure time, and close relationships. These needs are important to everybody and do not go away after a head injury.

I was lucky to find T work in a place founded by people under similar circumstances. They realize how important it is for T to have a job to enhance her self-esteem. She sorts auto parts and works three mornings a week. The insurance company actually supplements the paycheck she receives from her employer, but she doesn't know this. T feels important and worthwhile going to work. She punches a time clock and on payday, we take her check to the bank. She signs it, and I sign underneath because her writing has not progressed very far. When the bank teller hands T the money, her smile reflects her sense of pride.

WHEN PARENTS CAN NO LONGER CARE FOR THE INJURED CHILD

Many children will grow into adults who will never be able to care for themselves. Many of the brain-injured children are in otherwise good health with good insurance plans, so the prognosis is for a long and healthy life, never mind the brain injury. Parents worry about what will happen to the children when they are no longer able to care for them.

Discussing these issues with other mothers moved me to take action to ensure a future for T when I will not be able to care for her. It prompted me to set up trust funds and investments for her. Her sister Renee said that when I can no longer care for T, she will get a house where she could have a place built for T to live and she will supervise the caregivers. More information about estate planning is contained in Section III.

OTHER PEOPLE'S REACTIONS TO A TRAUMATIC BRAIN INJURY

Some of the mothers I interviewed talked about problems with taking their child with a brain injury out in public. I found that it is within my power to set the tone for peoples' reactions and to make strangers feel more at ease by being matter-of-fact about things. I discovered this when I took T to a restaurant. While we were going in, I conversed with her, smiled at people, and displayed a positive attitude. I could see acceptance reflected in other people.

Some of my friends do not speak about T. I think it is because they are uneasy about the topic and don't know what to say. Others ask automatically how she is doing; I always have the feeling they want only a positive response. Some parents seem skittish or edgy around me. I suspect it is because it makes them realize their own vulnerability or that of their children. After all, they are human and something like T's accident could happen to them. Our family dentist said, "This is something that happens to other people, not people we know."

ASSISTANCE FOR THE PATIENT

Patients often need special education placement for several years after a brain injury. This specialized coaching can be extremely helpful in recovering some intellectual ability. The public schools now have a category within special education for brain injury, with specially trained teachers to help this type of student.

Photographs or video feedback can be helpful. Making a video tape of the patient in physical therapy might be useful when viewed later in time. This can enhance the self-esteem of the patients when they realize the progress that they have made. Keeping a scrapbook or journal is also a creative outlet. These can serve as records of progress. T has an ongoing scrapbook created with the aid of others. It helps remind her of the things she has done and places she has been.

One thing T particularly enjoys is going out with her caregivers. They take her shopping, to concerts, to get her nails done, or they engage in other forms of recreation. She enjoys the stimulation of being around crowds. This is rather ironic since other people with brain injuries may find this kind of stimulation overwhelming. T's week is packed full of activities and a typical week is as follows:

- Monday: T works in the morning and has arts and crafts in the afternoon.

- Tuesday: I work, so Brenda is with her from 1:00 to 10:00 PM. They do things that are fun and often go to the movies.

- Wednesday: T works in the morning and works with her speech therapist on the Mini-Mo speech machine in the afternoon.

- Thursday: T has music therapy in the morning, and we spend the afternoon together. We might have lunch out or go to a dental or medical appointment.

- Friday: Total Transportation picks T up to take her to work. After work, twice a month, they transport her to Renee's house so she can spend quality time with her sister while the children are in school. She comes home at 4:30 PM and at 5:00 PM we are on our way to her swimming session.

- Saturday: I work and Dienna is with her from 1:00 to 10:00 PM. They shop, have pedicures, go on picnics, and work on T's scrapbook. It gives Chuck and me time away in the evening for a "date night."
- Sunday: T attends the special church program.
- Once a month, T spends Friday and Saturday night at Michelle's Farm.

Her week is busy and chocked full of activities. I believe this lends "quality" to her life.

PROFESSIONALS

Throughout my dealings with the professionals, I was constantly asked what I wanted for T. I always knew that I wanted "quality of life" for her and, as I stated earlier, I think we have found that according to our own definition.

The mothers I interviewed felt that the professionals did not have a good understanding of what families need. Many mothers desperately need assistance of some sort and professionals just aren't knowledgeable on what resources are available or helpful. Mothers commented they feel that they know more than the professionals because the professionals live with the patients eight hours a day, as opposed to the mothers' twenty-four-hour shift.

The professional's misperception is complicated by the fact that some significant others engage in what is called "command performance syndrome." One study found that significant others tended to appear relatively normal in the presence of the patient and health care professionals, choosing not to display their actual feelings (Spordone, Kral, Gerald, and Katz 1984, 183–185). Although they may not be denying their feelings, they are not actually forthcoming about how they feel in front of professionals. Under these circumstances, professionals may not really realize the trauma they are experiencing.

A similar study addressed the medical professionals' lack of understanding of the changes within the person with a head injury and communication gaps between members of the medical profession (Spanbock 1987, 12–14). These factors lead to a lack of information for the family. If the medical community bridged the existing gap in medical knowledge as well as communicated better among themselves, the families would probably have more of the information they desire.

Another study that echoed what I heard concerned over-protectiveness, financial problems, and emotional strain. It suggested increased community services, career guidance, and social networks to aid the head injured patients (Karpman, Wolfe, & Vargo 1986, 28–33). The mothers also felt that once their children finished with rehabilitation, there were no adequate outlets for them if they were not functioning high enough to be mainstreamed with society.

Misunderstandings can easily occur between professionals and family members simply through word choice. Professionals should be careful when using the word "recovery." While they generally mean "improvement," the family members often perceive the word "recovery" as meaning a "return to normal" (Zarski, DePompei, & Zack 1988, 31–41).

While psychological counseling is helpful to families, it does not protect the family from experiencing the pain and suffering of grief and loss; however, it does help them cope with the situation. Several mothers found counseling to be helpful. I believe we need therapists who specialize in working with the grief family members face when having a family member suffer a brain injury.

DENIAL

Denial is a psychological defense mechanism that helps people cope with and adjust to a situation that is too uncomfortable or painful to accept. Instead the person rejects it and insists that it is not true despite what may be overwhelming evidence. The person may deny the reality of the unpleasant fact altogether (simple denial), admit the fact but deny its seriousness (minimization), or admit both the fact and seriousness but deny responsibility (transference).

At first, the implications of a brain injury are just too overwhelming to consider. I know that I was in denial for some time. I couldn't accept the fact that T wasn't just going to wake up and be the perky, energetic thirteen-year old who was in the accident. When the medical staff gave me pamphlets and brochures about traumatic brain injury, I thought, "These aren't for me," and stuck them in a drawer without looking at them. I felt like I was in a fog for months. The days and weeks ran together, and it was hard to keep track of time. After about two months, I began to emerge from the fog. I suddenly wanted to know all I could about brain injury and started reading everything I could find. I think this is when I emerged from denial and started taking control of my life. I viewed knowledge and information as a form of control. Dick stayed in a form of denial until he died. That was how he coped. While I wanted T to come home and live with us, he did not and denial allowed him to believe that T was better off living in a rehab facility because they could help her recover. He was holding out for a higher level of "recovery."

Denial can be helpful initially but if it continues too long, it can inhibit progress and restrain people from getting on with their lives.

STAGES OF DEALING WITH THE INJURY

As families move through shock, professionals should help them understand that recovery may not be complete. Active mourning needs to take place. Because the patient still lives, there is an extension of the mourning process and prolonged sorrow.

There is a study on the subject which delineates several stages in the process of dealing with a brain injury (Lezak 1986, 242–247):

- In the beginning stage, psychologists need to help family members observe the patient's condition accurately. Denial is prevalent.

- In the second stage, families tend to be more receptive to the idea that recovery will not be complete.

- In the third stage, family members need to disassociate from the invested attitudes and ties that characterized earlier relationships with the patient. At this stage, the family is beginning to be conscious of their desire to escape a burdensome, unrewarding, and restructuring situation. They need to develop coping mechanisms and ways to manage stress.

- In the fourth stage, the family sees the patient as a person who is different from the person they knew before or as "a person they neither raised nor chose."

- In the fifth stage, active mourning takes place. However, mourning for a living person is "socially" unacceptable. Unlike a death, there are no institutionalized rituals for this mourning. It is an isolating and often secretive sorrowing prolonged by the presence of the patient. This is the most difficult of all mourning situations, where the lost person still "lives."

- In the sixth stage, the family reaches emotional detachment. The family must preserve health, sanity, and morale as much as possible. The dependent patient's welfare depends on the well-being of the family. Family members may be able to endure a life of self-denial for a few days or weeks, but no one can endure a regiment of emotional and social deprivation indefinitely without becoming ill, emotionally disturbed, or both.

Therefore, it is extremely important that the family develop coping mechanisms, which include respite, stress reduction techniques, and utilization of the resources that are available to help them get on with their lives.

GRIEVING

The grief families experience does not follow the standard grieving model because there is not a death. The family has lost a part of the person they once knew. Families also grieve for the part of themselves they lose because of the loss of that part of the child.

Dr. Phillip Barry, who was head of the facility in New York where T was a patient, has done a great deal of research on the process families go through. He wrote that the head-injured victim and the family share the long process of recovery. Their ability to deal with this difficult process will ultimately affect each member of the family. In order to reach a stage where a person can accept the loss that has occurred, grief must be experienced. He believes grief is both a reaction to loss and an important aspect of recovery. He outlined four stages (Barry 1987, 449). The first stage is shock and denial. The second stage is anxiety and panic. The third is anger, sometimes experienced as guilt. The last stage is one of depression. He believes mourning is a natural part of the grief process. It may seem all is lost and there is nothing left to recover. The future for the injured family member is hopeless with nothing to live for. He says this outlook is as irrational as expectations for total recovery.

I frequently recall what the resident physician told me in the early weeks of T's brain injury when he said "the abnormal will become normal." I couldn't begin to accept what he said at the time, but now I understand. Humankind is resilient and able to adjust. We go on to incorporate those abnormalities and integrate them into our normal daily life. My own mourning was a very solitary experience. What I came to realize is that I not only lost my energetic thirteen-year old daughter in the car accident that night, but I also lost a piece of myself. While I still have T, she is changed and so am I. I also lost the hopes and dreams that I had for her. The dreams I had for T were that she would find love, have a family, and I would have grandchildren from her. I had also relished her dream of being a veterinarian. I have mourned and grieved over my lost dreams for T. As in many families, my own family members were at different parts of the grieving continuum at any particular time. Therefore, we would each try to console one another from a very different point of view. For example, Dick was in denial and was angry when I was being nurturing and needed consoling. Dick could not console me at that point because of his denial and anger. This caused stress between us.

The classical grieving model has another phase: acceptance. Acceptance can also be a phase of the process. Acceptance is alluded to, searched for, and sometimes found. Acceptance leads to an understanding of the permanence of the situation but does not always imply finding answers to why tragedies such as brain injuries occur. As families begin to accept the idea that the patient's recovery will never be complete, coping mechanisms need to be developed because the patient's welfare depends on the well being of the family, especially that of the mother. The family also needs to look at the frustrations that trigger stress. The fact remains that although brain injury is a continuum as far as healing is concerned, the patient will never be the same as before the accident. This is often what is so frustrating for the caregivers and family.

CHAPTER 3:
IMPACT ON FAMILY

The impact on the family can be very difficult. One of the most difficult things for me is that I could always fix things for T with a bandage or kiss; if she had a quarrel with a friend, I could talk with her. Frequently I now feel so helpless. You can never change what happened, but you can understand traumatic brain injury, your options, and take steps to adapt along the way. Your family will feel out of control, so it is important to take time to step back, share feelings, and consider how you can support each other. If you look, you can find resources in your community to help.

A head injury changes not only the patient's life, but the lives of all the family members as well. This change could take an unhealthy turn if the family, as a whole, tries to resume life as though nothing has happened. Families need to establish new routines that take into account the needs of the member with a head injury. One study of families with a member with a brain injury showed that the amount and type of stress felt by family members depended on their position within the family. It became evident that the family member displaying the closest relationship to the patient experienced the most stress. The study also showed that stress interfered with that member's daily performance of activities. Mothers are usually in the closest position and most vulnerable to this position of stress (Reese 1983, 72–77).

Family relationships shift over time as roles and responsibilities change with the injury. Such shifts present special problems in communication. Other relatives (such as siblings, children, and grandparents) or friends may be so uncomfortable with the situation that they may deny the illness. They may feel overwhelmed and cut off communication at a time when they really need each other's support. If the strains are too great, a family member might shut down, feeling hopeless, isolated, and trapped. Sometimes relatives fret over minor issues while holding back painful news, angry feelings, or resentments.

When you identify your fears (death of your child, loss of freedom), you're less likely to express them inappropriately or take them out on others. You can help jump-start essential, good communication by:

- Identifying your own needs

- Recognizing that life goes on

- Learning to send "I" messages: "I feel angry when I have to take the child to the doctor by myself" or "I feel great that you helped by taking the child to the doctor"

If you use these approaches, you'll model good communication skills for everyone, gain a sense of control, and take ownership of your feelings at the same time.

After families begin to accept the idea that the patient's recovery will never be complete, they need to develop coping and stress reduction strategies. If the family is not okay, the patient will not be okay. I know I am always looking out for T's welfare and planning what she can do next so she doesn't get bored. Things often conflict with my schedule, and I am always juggling my calendar to accommodate her needs. In addition to coping with stress, the family needs to look at the frustrations that trigger stress. One trigger is that although brain injury is a continuum as far as healing is concerned, the patient will never be the same as before the accident. This is often what is so frustrating for the family: The family is changed forever.

Denial also enters into family dynamics and functioning. One study showed that parents showing poor emotional adjustment to their children's head injury were more inclined to use denial as a coping strategy (Tarter 1990, 15–22). While denial can be useful in the initial stages of an injury, if it persists, psychological intervention can be useful. Another study found denial as a major obstacle to successful adaptation in the family with a member with a head injury. The study also found that rehabilitation professionals do not have enough information about what kind of response is most beneficial for the family (Ridley 1990, 555–561). I felt that if I tried hard enough, T would be okay. Maybe that was like a child's unrealistic concept of control. I have a friend who had a sister in a coma for years because of a traumatic brain injury. Neither the patient's mother nor her four sisters visited her because they said they "couldn't stand to see her that way." My friend was the only one who visited her. This is an extreme case of denial. The whole situation for the family is complicated because, as discussed previously, all family members are in different stages at the same time and may try to console the others from very different points of view.

MOTHERS

As I interviewed the mothers, I realized that mothers are the nurturers and primary caregivers. They are responsible for making the family function. This is often overwhelming for the mother, and studies show the emotional health of the caregiver is critical in balancing the functions of the family (Zarski, DePompei, & Zack 1988: 31–41). Loneliness and isolation are not only issues for the patient but also for the mother who experiences this because her focus is on the family and the child with the brain injury. As I mentioned earlier, a relationship with another person is important so that the person with a head injury feels loved. Fortunately or unfortunately, the loving must often come from the mother alone, which can make her even more isolated.

Another facet of my experience with T, which I now understand, is how her father's role influenced me. I have always assumed the primary nurturing role in our family structure. As my awareness of this became clearer, I realized a need to share this nurturing role with her father because I felt so lonely and isolated. Some of the other mothers I interviewed expressed a similar need for support from the fathers. Support groups were sometimes helpful; yet most of the time I felt attendees had no idea of what I was experiencing.

SIBLINGS

Siblings often feel a sense of neglect because so much attention is focused on the injured child. Pat, one of the mothers I interviewed, said her other children virtually went to high school on their own because she was so preoccupied with Marcus. Her daughter never brought friends home because Marcus would make loud grunting noises and roll around on the floor and this embarrassed her. She has a lot of hatred toward her mother for ignoring her. Pat's son never played sports because he was filling in for his mother as caregiver for his brother when she had other things to do. This sort of neglect needs to be avoided.

I think what happened with T's sister Renee was that some old memories began to surface. I had Renee when I was young, and I needed to work at the time. Dick was on a co-op program and worked only six months of the year. Dick's mom helped me take care of Renee because I was working. When T was born, I had the luxury of staying home. I later realized that Renee, understandably, felt that she didn't get the same attention from me as I gave to T. When T was injured, my time and focus were again on her. Renee was living away from home by then, but I am sure she felt as if I had placed her on the back burner once again.

FATHERS

Dick was definitely involved in T's care. But he placed most of his energy into lawyers, insurance companies, and other necessary but practical concerns. I found it true that many of the fathers took care of these issues, while the mother took responsibility for the care and nurturing issues. When there is only one parent, all of these duties can be overwhelming. Dick also worried about T's future, and wanted "the most for the dollar" for her. He had a good heart, and I think, like many men, was practical at the expense of his feelings. I tried to talk about my pain and although he was close to tears several times, he tightened up against his own feelings. Most of the other mothers I interviewed reported their husbands kept an emotional distance.

I think men in our culture want to "fix" whatever is wrong. With a head injury, there is a feeling of helplessness. Dick continued to be angry at the legal system, also. The young lady who caused the accident spent only a few months in detention because there was not room for her. She was cited for driving without a license since the accident and suffered no consequences. It seemed that Dick wanted justice, but I was not sure how justice applied since it would not bring T back. At other times, Dick's goal orientation seemed to get in the way. However, like all of us, he did the best he could in an extremely difficult situation.

OTHER RELATIVES

Dick's mother was a great source of support for him, and she was often at the hospital or traveling with us to Virginia or New York. Unfortunately, she did not have the same effect on me, and that was probably due somewhat to the mother-in-law/daughter-in-law thing. I always had the feeling I wasn't quite the girl she wanted Dick to marry. But then again, I don't think any woman would have been really good enough for her Dick. Early on in my marriage, I fretted over what I could do to make her like me and finally realized that it was her issue, not mine.

What happens in most families is that the person closest to the victim is affected the most, financial struggles impact the families, and these and other concerns set the stage for stress to overwhelm them.

CHAPTER 4:
STRESSES ASSOCIATED
WITH A TRAUMATIC BRAIN
INJURY

While working on my dissertation, I did many literature searches on the mother's experience with her child's traumatic brain injury and came up with nothing. I thought at the time that the lack of information was perhaps because the number of people who had sustained and survived one of these injuries had only recently greatly increased. I supposed this specialized care was a relatively new circumstance due to the accelerated advancement of medical technology and the latest educational and governmental requirements. I thought that perhaps the research and literature in this field might just be starting and would be available to help mothers in a couple of years. However, doing a literature search in 2006 returned no significant new information in helping the family deal with a brain injury. This was one of the motivating factors for writing this book. I want to help families understand and cope with the stress and trauma they are experiencing. While there is a lot of self-help information available on stress and dealing with stress, the solutions suggested are like a drop of water when we are dealing with the ocean. Some suggestions are fine for everyday working people, executives, and the overwhelmed, but they are fairly insufficient when you consider what the family dealing with a child with a traumatic brain injury is experiencing. The information is general, and you have to wade through pages of it to find something that is appropriate for your situation. Consequently, the need for this information and inadequacy of what is available added to my desire to share what I have learned.

Reflecting on my experience with regard to stress and time management, I discovered that I needed to continually prioritize my activities and take time to nurture myself. I do this by engaging in hobbies and interests that bring me peace and joy. Prioritizing activities makes sure the most important things get done, and time for myself helps me to return to T somewhat replenished.

The things that have given me the most peace and solace on a day-to-day basis are meditation, yoga, and journaling. I meditated and kept a journal before T's accident, and I don't know how I would have survived without these tools. Meditation helps me to calm my mind and spirit; journaling helps me to express my feelings in a safe environment. It is almost a purging of emotions or a way of transferring the emotional feeling to paper. I took up yoga a year ago, which is wonderful for releasing stress and tension in the body as well as helping to clear the mind. All of these activities help me to return to T renewed.

This is not to say I don't struggle everyday with the time management element in the form of priorities, because I do. On top of that, I need to feel that I have done everything possible, both for T and myself. It took me a long time and many struggles to realize how to do it. Even now, at this moment when I am sitting in my office at home working on this book, the sound of "mom," over and over again interrupts the sounds of music coming from the room where T is practicing with her music therapist. Music therapy is only an hour in our house, but I view it as an hour when I have time to myself to write, read, think, and be. I hesitate to use the word be "free," because I don't think I will really ever be totally free, which Chuck pointed out to me recently. Despite arranging free time for me and my husband, my thoughts often wander back to T. It is not unlike the feeling a new parent has when she leaves her newborn with someone else.

On top of this, there are the psycho-social aspects experienced by the patient; they often feel isolated, lonely, and worthless. Therefore, a relationship with another person is extremely important, and it is often the mother filling this role. Pat, one of the mothers I interviewed, said that in the evening when things quieted down and she might have time to read or relax, she often found herself with her son because she felt he might be lonely.

Ironically, as it is for the victim, isolation is a major stressor for the caregiver as well. This is why respite care is so vital. It's also important for the mother to maintain as normal a life as possible as far as interests and career are concerned. Obtaining quality help is difficult. For some people, the more financially secure they are, the easier it is to get quality help. This is unfortunate for people who don't have the means. In my particular case, the scheduled monthly respite care at the farm and help from T's other angels give me time. Maximizing my inner life has been a "godsend." For me that means yoga and meditation. For someone else it may be organized religion or exercise.

There are many things that occur day in and day out in the lives of a family with a member with a brain injury. All of these contribute to the stress experienced by each and every member. Because of the long-lasting implications of living in a state of continual stress, it is extremely important for members to take whatever measures necessary to decrease the stress and discover ways to cope with it.

Chapter 5:
Anatomy of stress

Stress is one of the circumstances I find most difficult to deal with. It bombards the family who has a child with a traumatic brain injury. It is part of the continuum and is always there. As I've pointed out, the mother most often becomes the primary caregiver for the child and, therefore, the one who can be most overwhelmed by the situation. The bottom line is that unless the mother can manage the stress, everyone will suffer because she is often the one responsible for effective family functioning. As the saying goes, "If Mama isn't happy, nobody is happy."

As I previously stated, when I did my dissertation very little information was available to help cope with the stress of having a child with a brain injury. It is my goal to provide some focused and structured information to help families. Stress is a fact of life for everyone, but for our families we are totally immersed in it, cannot get away from it, and must learn to manage it. Since the people reading this book may be at different levels of sophistication in dealing with stress, I will start with some basics.

WHAT IS STRESS?

Here is the best definition I have found: Stress is the psychological and physiological reaction that takes place when one perceives an imbalance in the level of demands and one's capacity to meet those demands. This happens to every family who has a child with a brain injury. The term "stress" was coined in the 1950's by Dr. Hans Selye, a physiologist who borrowed the term from physicists, and used it in the biological sense we know today. Dr. Selye defined stress as "the body's nonspecific response to any demand." He proposed there were hormones that came from the hypothalamus, the pituitary, and the adrenal glands and these could also effect how the immune system works. The concept was revolutionary for that time.

We generally explain stress as the "flight or fight" response that is innate in every person. This goes back to when man was in primitive societies and would be faced with a life-threatening situation; he would have to decide whether to fight or flee whenever a threat was posed. The autonomic nervous system takes over and increases our stress chemicals (adrenaline, cortisol, and noradrenalin). The heart rate increases, blood pressure elevates, blood is shunted from the stomach to the muscles, muscle tension is increased, breathing quickens, pupils dilate, perspiration increases, oxygen intake increases, glucose and fatty acids are mobilized, and blood coagulants to aid in clotting are released.

Barb Schoen, in her article *Families and Disability*, lists the following factors that influence your level of stress (Schoen 2007, 4):

- Whether your caregiving is voluntary. If you feel you had no choice in taking on the responsibilities, the chances are greater that you will experience strain, distress, and resentment.

- Your relationship with the care recipient. Sometimes people care for another with the hope of healing a relationship. If healing does not occur, you may feel regret and discouragement.

- Your coping abilities. How you coped with stress in the past predicts how you will cope now. Identify your current coping strengths so that you can build on them.

- Your caregiving situation. Some caregiving situations are more stressful than others. For example, caring for a person with dementia is often more stressful than caring for someone with a physical limitation.

- Whether support is available.

WHAT ARE THE PHYSICAL SIGNS OF STRESS?

When under continual stress, people become more prone to frequent illness. Some of the physical signs include headaches, backaches, muscle fatigue, changes in appetite, insomnia, oversleeping, accident-proneness, dry mouth, stiff neck, irregular heartbeat, hyperventilation, cold hands, butterflies, eye strain, gritted teeth, indigestion, and physical exhaustion. In addition, stress compromises the immune system, making one more susceptible to colds, flu, and other illnesses.

WHAT ARE THE EMOTIONAL/BEHAVIORAL SIGNS OF STRESS?

People exhibit many different behaviors. These include apathy or the "blahs," crying episodes, sudden angry outbursts, mood swings, feelings of restlessness, inability to concentrate, feeling preoccupied, increase in absences, tardiness, marked differences in grooming habits, withdrawal from relationships at work, avoiding things and/or doing things to extremes, such as alcohol consumption, gambling, spending sprees, and sexual promiscuity. Emotions are constantly with us, shifting the way we see the world.

WHAT ARE THE MOST COMMON EMOTIONAL DISORDERS RELATED TO STRESS?

Emotional disorders related to stress include alcoholism and drug abuse, depression, suicide, marital and family problems, and sexual dysfunction.

WHAT ARE THE PHYSICAL DISORDERS RELATED TO STRESS?

Some experts say the majority of illnesses are stress-related. These include coronary heart disease and heart attack, high blood pressure and hypertension, diabetes, allergies, eczema, asthma, chronic bronchitis, colitis, kidney disease, sinusitis, cancer, stomach upset, and infectious and inflammatory diseases.

WHEN IS STRESS GOOD AND WHEN IS IT BAD?

Good stress, or eustress, is what motivates you; it provides stimulation and challenges. Deadlines get us going. But when there is too much stress, it is overwhelming and signals the body's stress response.

SCIENTIFIC DOCUMENTATION THAT STRESS CAN MAKE YOU SICK.

A book titled, *The Balance Within, the Science Connecting Health and Emotions*,
by Esther Sternberg, is about the science connecting health and emotions. Dr.
Sternberg is a biomedical researcher and rheumatologist. She explains how stress
can trigger hormonal responses in the body to make you sick and, conversely,
how people can recover by consciously choosing to get well (Sternberg 2001,
109–132). This book is informative and interesting because Dr. Sternberg comes
from not only a very sound scientific research background, but she experienced
both the psychological and physiological burnout as well as the recovery about
which she writes. I also found a lot of information from the following Web site
(http://speakingoffaith.publicradio.org/programs/stress/undex.shtml) and have
summarized this information in the following paragraphs:

What did Dr. Sternberg discover that is different from what Dr. Seyle knew in
the 1950s? Dr. Sternberg's work revolved around the intricate network that exists
between the immune system and the brain. This network allows the two systems
to continuously and rapidly signal each other. Chemicals produced by immune
cells signal the brain, and the brain in turn sends chemical signals to restrain the
immune system. These same chemical signals also affect behavior and the
response to stress.

Dr. Sternberg explained that something happens between the time you're
faced with a threat and the time your body physiologically responds to it. What
happens is your perception of the event interprets and colors the way your body
responds to it. Therefore, your memory plays a big role in how you perceive an
event, which could be threatening, stressful, or happy, depending on what your
past experiences are. For example, one person might view the boss approaching
her desk as a positive experience if she has a good working relationship with the
boss and finds that the boss often asks her for suggestions about managing the
workplace. Another person might view it as a negative experience if the boss only

comes to her desk when she is going to be criticized. The stimulus of the boss approaching the desk is going to affect each person differently depending on what has happened in the past.

People from all walks of life who need to make rapid, frequent decisions or perform under pressure learn to make the most of the stress response by using it to maximize their performance. Furthermore, these people also learn or are trained to lower their stress response because they know how to react. Examples of such individuals might be doctors in emergency rooms, lawyers, airplane pilots, executives, secretaries, and homemakers. These people have learned to deal with many tasks at the same time.

Families with a child with a traumatic brain injury may learn over time how to better manage the stresses of caring for the child. When I returned to school to get my Ph.D., I knew that many people would see the pressures of being a student as a stress-provoking situation. I saw it as something I could control and a process to achieve a life-long goal. Although it was rough at times, I knew I was in control and could always focus on achieving my goal; and having an achievable goal was important since the part of my life involving T was so unpredictable.

Perception is vital in dealing with stress. Dr. Sternberg says it is the way our memory perceives an event which determines whether or not it is threatening. She believes that if we can change our perception or construct a new memory, then we can change our reaction and decrease the stress response. However, it takes time to construct a new memory or habit. You have to practice it over and over again, sometimes up to fifty times before it becomes routine. It has to become a habit.

Dr. Sternberg adds it is not the stress itself that makes you sick but rather the hormones and nerve pathways that are activated by stress (Sternberg 2001, 109–132). When stress becomes chronic, these hormones change the response of the immune system, making it less able to fight disease. She thinks these findings could have profound effects on the treatments for nervous system and immune system illnesses. Moreover, she thought it substantiated that our state of mind can influence how well we resist or recover from infectious or inflammatory diseases. Stress can make you sick because you have an overactive immune system. It is very important to turn off the immune system cells. When you're chronically stressed and pumping out hormones, your immune cells will be bathed in these cells and not be available when you are exposed to infections.

Dr. Sternberg was writing an article, which is the basis for her book, while her mother was dying of breast cancer. She told her mother that the stress response could make one sick. Her mother pressured her to take the article further and argued that if we know that stress can make us sick, we could assume that loving and believing can help us be well. Dr. Sternberg resisted doing this until she herself burned out, became ill with arthritis, and was forced to stop what she was doing in order to rest and recover. Then she decided to write *The Balance Within*.

CHANGE

Another thing Dr. Sternberg talks about in her research is the novelty of a new situation or change. She says there are responses that take place in the brain when change occurs. This is not really new, and is something we've known for awhile. In 1967 Dr. Thomas Holmes, a psychiatrist, and Richard Rahe, a Navy scientist, introduced the Social Readjustment Rating Scale, also known as the Holmes-Rahe stress scale. The scale consists of forty-three events, ranging from the death of a spouse to minor violations of the law that can indicate a susceptibility to some illnesses. Most of the top stressors on this scale have to do with change, regardless of whether it is a positive or negative change.

Those who are critical of this scale argue that some people respond differently from others to these life events; therefore, the rating scale is not appropriate for all, even though it does demonstrate the fact that change is stressful. Being the caretaker of a child with a brain injury almost tops the scale of stress level.

PREMATURE AGING

An article in *Scientific American (11/30/04)* by Elissa S. Epel of the University of California at San Francisco showed that stress may take a toll on your health by affecting the strands of DNA on the ends of chromosomes. She recruited thirty-nine mothers of chronically ill children and compared them to mothers with healthy children. She found the mothers with sick children had shorter telomeres, which play an important role in cellular aging. Moreover, the difference between the stressed mothers and the control group was equivalent to nearly a decade of additional aging. Further, Dr. Epel says, "The new findings suggest a cellular mechanism for how chronic stress may cause premature onset of disease. Chronic stress appears to have the potential to shorten the life of cells, at least immune cells."

Understanding stress, what it does, and finding ways to cope are important steps for the well being of the whole family.

Chapter 6:
Ways of coping and
managing stress

I realize that having a child with a traumatic brain injury is an all-encompassing, life-altering experience. It is the worst thing a parent ever faces, and some refer to it as the "never-ending nightmare." You have no time for yourself, and mothers in particular end up devoting themselves to their injured child. To survive and do what is best for your child, you need to find a way to cope with the trying circumstances and escape the situation. I don't think anyone can get away without guilt. However, if you understand that by pushing yourself to the max you can break down and get sick, it makes you feel less guilty when you take time for yourself. Dr. Sternberg discovered that we can consciously choose to improve our health. Sometimes you need to shut down and reboot, just like your computer. Barb Schoen, in her article *Families and Disability*, lists the following effects of care giving on health and well being (Schoen 2007, 2):

- Sleep deprivation

- Poor eating habits

- Failure to exercise

- Failure to stay in bed when ill

- Postponement of or failure to make medical appointments

- Caregivers over 66 are 63% more likely to die than peers

At times, you may need to seek professional help because there could be a chemical imbalance taking place within the body that only a physician can accurately diagnose and treat. For example, after my husband died, I went into a deep depression and it was the realization that I needed to be there for T that finally motivated me to get professional help. In that case, medication helped me to recover. The self-help stress industry is a multi-million dollar business, and it is going strong. Just go into any bookstore and peruse the shelves of books written about stress and coping. Although all those pages contain information that may be pertinent to certain people who are stressed, they do not begin to tap into the kind of stress that is experienced by the parent of a child with a brain injury. It is like trying to empty the Great Lakes with a cup; it just doesn't work. I found a lot of useful information from the following Web site (http://zenhabits.net/2007/09/simple-living-manifesto-72-ideas-to-simplify-your-life/) and have summarized them here:

Take Control

Many of us deal with stress in the wrong way. A 2005 survey by the advocacy group Mental Health America found many people deal with chronic stress by watching television, skipping exercise, and foregoing healthy foods. Also, people find comfort in alcohol and drugs. None of these is helpful because they keep you from the things that can help reduce the effects of stress. Barb Schoen, in her article *Families and Disability*, lists the following in identifying personal barriers and taking responsibility for your own care (Schoen 2007, 3):

- Many times, attitudes and beliefs form personal barriers that stand in the way of caring for yourself.

- Not taking care of yourself may be a lifelong pattern, with taking care of others an easier option.

- However, as a family caregiver you must ask yourself, "What good will I be to the person I care for if I become ill? If I die?"

- Do you feel you have to prove that you are worthy of the care recipient's affection?

- Do you think you are being selfish if you put your needs first?

- Is it frightening to think of your own needs? What is the fear about?

- Do you have trouble asking for what you need? Do you feel inadequate if you ask for help? Why?

It is extremely important that you productively manage your time and life. You can take control of your life in many ways. First and foremost is to learn about traumatic brain injury. The more information you have, the more you feel in control. The resource section of this book is filled with listings of where to obtain information. Remember when I mentioned the doctor's comment about the abnormal becoming normal? I dismissed him at the time as I wasn't ready to hear it but later I realized he did know what he was saying. It did take time for things to feel normal. When you get used to the day-to-day management of your child, you can consider more in-depth planning. Initially this is scary when you look into the face of the future, but it can help you regain control when you can look ahead.

Identify the challenges you face. Take stock of what you want, need, and are capable of accomplishing. It's okay to have wishes, as well as fears and anger. These are a natural part of the process. When you plan carefully, you may find that something you thought was impossible might be possible. Understand your own coping process. It takes time to accept what has happened. People stay in denial for years. Adjusting to change is a challenge. Sometimes it means managing with less money, fighting for entitlements, filling out forms, or learning to use assistive devices that may require new skills. Understanding what approach works best for you can help. Change your attitude, simplify your life, join a support group, and learn all you can.

Barb Schoen, in her article *Families and Disability*, lists several steps you can take to manage your stress (Schoen 2007, 5):

- Recognize warning signs early. These might include irritability, sleep problems, and forgetfulness. Know your own warning sign and act to make changes. Don't wait until you are overwhelmed.

- Identify sources of stress. Ask yourself, "What is causing stress for me?" Sources of stress might be too much to do, family disagreements, feeling of inadequacy, and inability to say no.

- Identify what you can and cannot change. Remember, we can only change ourselves; we cannot change another person.

- Take action. Taking some action to reduce stress gives us back a sense of control. Stress reducers can be simple activities like walking and other forms of exercise, gardening, meditation, or having coffee with a friend. Identify some stress reducers that work for you.

CONTROL YOUR ATTITUDE

The first thing that you can control is your attitude. Dr. Sternberg discovered that something happens between the time you're faced with a threat and your body responds physiologically. That's where memory comes in. Your perception of the event determines how your body responds to it. If your body reacts with the "stress response" and floods your body with chemicals, that can have a negative effect and wear down your immune system if it happens repeatedly. What you can do is teach your body the "relaxation response," and establish a new habit. When something happens that evokes the stress response, here's what you can do: Stop. Take a few deep breaths. Then count to twenty, say a prayer, recite a mantra, have a place of solitude you can retreat to in your memory, or develop some ritual you elicit when needed. Find a technique that works for you. If you call on the same technique each time stress strikes, you will establish a new habit and the familiarity will evoke a "relaxation response" instead of a "stress response." Your memory will automatically take over. I've always liked the first part of the Serenity Prayer which I interpret as attitude:

Serenity Prayer
Source Unknown

God grant me the serenity
to accept the things I cannot change;
courage to change the things I can;
and wisdom to know the difference.

I believe going back to school to get a Ph.D. was the best thing I could do at that point in time because it gave me some control in my life. The only way I could manage my time was to prioritize my activities, live in the moment, and focus on the project in which I was engaged. I recently went to a yoga seminar and the teachers stressed being in the moment, saying the only moment we are sure of is the one we are in. It seems to me that is what I was doing, and it was very helpful. Another writing that quickly summarizes the value of attitude follows:

Attitude
Source Unknown

The longer I live, the more I realize the impact of attitude on life. Attitude, to me, is more important than facts. It is more important than the past, than education, than money, than circumstances, than failures, than successes, than what other people think, say, or do. It is more important than appearance, giftedness, or skill. It will make or break a company, a church, a home. The remarkable thing is we have a choice every day regarding the attitude we will embrace for that day.

We cannot change our past. We cannot change the fact that people will act in a certain way. We cannot change the inevitable. The only thing we can do is play on the one string we have, and that is our attitude. I am convinced that life is 10 percent what happens to me and 90 percent how I react to it. And so it is with you. We are in charge of our attitudes.

SIMPLIFY YOUR LIFE

The self-help industry has thousands of books about simplifying your life. Many espouse taking back your life through simplification because our possessions and lifestyles are too demanding and stressful. Many studies and statistics talk about how we are wrecking our lives, families, and the environment because of all the stuff we have and want. While there is a lot of truth to this, it's not what you want to hear when you're stressed to the max; what you need are some simple tips for simplifying your life.

Simplicity involves freeing your time, money, and energy so that you can pay more attention to what is important to you. Begin with the premise that your stress is exacerbated when you cannot find something. And when you are stressed, your memory doesn't work quite as well and it becomes easier to forget where you put something. One of the most useless time wasters is looking for what you can't find. This is the best reason to simplify: so that you can find what you need when you want it. By streamlining your life and reducing clutter, you're more apt to be able to locate important things because there will be less places for them to hide.

Often, one of the problems we experience is that we just have too much stuff to keep organized. So we have to figure out how to reduce what we have. Getting rid of things can be one of the most liberating things you do. Look for multiple ways to streamline your life and build more efficient habits and ways of doing things.

PARE DOWN AND STREAMLINE

There are several things you can do to pare down and streamline:

- **Organize methodically**. Cut through your stuff by regularly performing the clutter triage on one small area of your home at a time. For example, work on a single closet, a section of a room, or a storage area. Don't tackle the whole basement or attic. By choosing just one area for one de-junking session, and saving the rest for the next time, you'll do the job more thoroughly and you'll feel a greater sense of accomplishment. It might be your office, kitchen or bedroom. Examine your possessions and ask yourself if you really need each of them.

- **Get rid of extras**. Pay particular attention to getting rid of items that are useful, but not in the quantity you may have accumulated. For example, pots and pans. You certainly need them but do you need five saucepans or three frying pans? Other examples include: pencils, pens, radios, clocks, chairs, extension cords, lamps, luggage, and calendars.

- **Get rid of unused major appliances, furniture, and vehicles as soon as possible.** These can take up an enormous amount of space and inconvenience you. Use Craig's List (www.craigslist.org)—an online, local community of classifieds and forums for free, and in a relatively non-commercial environment. This is a great place to sell or give away things quickly and efficiently. Post your items and people will call to arrange the sale for cash. Also Freecycle (www.freecycle.org) is a Web site in which you can offer free goods to people in your area.

ORGANIZE

There are several ways in which you can get organized:

- **List things to do**. To aid organization, list all of the things you need to accomplish. Then review the list and ask which things you do not really need to do and cross them off the list.

- **Break down your projects into chunks, then to specific tasks, and then work on the tasks regularly.** Start every day with a list of tasks that you are working on. Write down your objectives and what you need to do to reach them. Crossing off tasks as you accomplish them reinforces your progress.

- **Handle paper once.** Designate a location for paperwork, bills, invitations and reminders, event tickets, and so on. Don't just stash them in one pile because they will get mislaid. Establish a system for the paperwork and medical information concerning your child with the brain injury and file everything in this one place. Post event tickets on a bulletin board. File event reminders in your calendar. Put bills in a "to do" folder. Most importantly, find a system that works for you and use it to assure that you will find what you need, when you need it.

- **Be prepared**. Prepare in advance the records, maps and appointment information you need when visiting a medical facility. Trying to locate the things you need when going to an appointment just before you walk out the door only adds to your stress and can make you late for your appointment. Include a diary to take to all medical appointments and include names of those nurses, doctors, etc. as well as recommendations they make. Dated diaries are a great help to recall when specific tests or procedures were done.

- **Revamp your clothing**. Did you know the 80/20 rule applies to your closet: You wear 20 percent of your clothes 80 percent of the time. What about that 80 percent you wear only 20 percent of the time? Another thing to consider is only having clothes that are easy to care for and comfortable. Get pieces that you can mix and match.

SAVE TIME

There are several steps you can take to save time:

- **Rearrange your work schedule**. If you have flex-time at work, consider starting work earlier to avoid rush hour traffic and give yourself more daylight hours off work. You'll get an earlier start on the day, and you might even have time in the afternoon to do errands before businesses close.

- **Anticipate and avoid peak times.** Use stores, streets, restaurants, services, and offices when others don't. The weekend is when many people are out. Save yourself time and aggravation by finding out and avoiding the peak time for any situation where you might get delayed. Think about what you need to do and try to do it during off-times.

- **Establish a regular, weekly shopping and errand day**. On your shopping day, do all your grocery, clothing, or supplies shopping at one time along with banking, and other errands. Your shopping day could be the time after work on a particular day in combination with a lunch period or time before or after work. A single shopping day consolidates both your time and trips, frees up other days of the week from the clutter of "running to the store," and reduces impulse buys. Getting errands done at a fixed time makes them more predictable and efficient.

- **Shop online**. Use on-line merchants to purchase some of the things you need. The great thing is you can do it any time of the day or night. Also, e-bay has some incredible bargains and merchandise.

- **Appearance**. Become low maintenance with a wash and wear hairstyle and minimal makeup.

- **Answering the phone, e-mail**. Screen your phone calls by using an answering machine. There may be some incoming calls you choose to ignore. Respond to e-mail every couple of days instead of daily; or if you have to update a number of people on a situation, develop a group e-mail list and send one e-mail for everyone.

- **Eliminate time commitments that don't matter to you.** Is there a commitment in your life right now that you are neglecting? If so, this neglect is a sign the commitment may not be important to you. Rethink the commitment and eliminate it if possible. Practice saying "no" so that this word is on your lips when asked to make a commitment you are not willing to accept.

- **Use a paper or computer-based organizer to write down your schedule, and names and phone numbers**. Keep track of the doctors and medical facilities you are working with. Record appointment times immediately and update your contacts list as needed. Portable, paper-based organizers can cost you less than ten dollars and be worth their weight in gold. Computer-based organizers can be updated quickly and backed up against loss. Many computer-based organizers can also be downloaded to a hand-held unit or printed on paper for portability.

- **Be on time**. Don't be late for appointments or deadlines because it raises your stress level and complicates your life. Anticipate problems, traffic jams, slow elevators, and getting a little lost. Plan to arrive at the building ten or fifteen minutes before your appointment if you are not familiar with its location. If you arrive early, you'll have time to use the restroom, get a drink of water, gather your thoughts, and present yourself in a calm, relaxed way at the appointment time. If you are late out of habit, mercilessly extinguish this habit. Don't put unnecessary stress on yourself by being late.

- **Use bits of time**. Every day has unavoidable delays, waits, and time between events. Use these bits of time for useful contemplation or work that can benefit you. Use the time spent waiting for the doctor or dentist to rework your shopping list. Do you have a regular commute on a bus or train? Read a book. Do you have a half hour before dinner? Do the "clutter purge" on one section of your desk or countertop or work on a hobby. Use bits of time to accomplish useful work that you would otherwise have to do some other time. Using bits of time also reminds you that you control your use your time, and waiting rooms or lines can serve a useful purpose.

- **Schedule time for relaxing and unwinding**. Set up a space in your house to meditate, practice yoga, read, do needlework, or just plain be. Most people cannot sustain a rigid time schedule for very long; they will deliberately or unconsciously sabotage it in order to get some time off. Worse yet, they may become ill because of a compromised immune system and pass the illness to other members of the family.

SUPPORT

It is important to have a good support system in place:

- **Social support networks**. Happiness experts have discovered that family, friends, pets, and community are the key to lasting happiness. And these are the resources that sustain us in hard times. It is easy to loose track of friends and associates at this time. When we are involved in our own crises, our friends are often out of sight and out of mind. My circle of friends was deteriorating for a couple of reasons. I did not have time to socialize and when I did run into people, it was awkward. I felt that many people just didn't know how to react to me. They either ignored me or treated me as if I were very fragile. I often felt they only wanted an "every thing's fine" kind of response. The best thing about being with my friend Helen, the woman who had a son with a brain injury, is that she lets me be myself; I don't have to put on a false face and pretend that things are all right. It is such a relief to just talk with someone who really understands what the situation is like, and not feel like I am complaining.

- **Make an appointment for quality time**. Saturday night is date night for Chuck and me. This has been very important for our relationship because we need to be sure we have some time together despite our busy schedules. The same thing can be done to keep up with other friends.

- **Entertain**. If you do want to keep up contacts with friends, you can plan more casual forms of entertaining that don't take up so much of your time. Instead of preparing a meal for company, invite people over for a potluck dinner. If you are going to a concert, play, or a game, invite people over for drinks before the event. That way you can get to see several friends at one time and maintain contact.

- **Join a support group**. Find a support group for parents with a child with a brain injury. It's a good way to not only share helpful information but to meet other parents in the same situation.

HOBBIES

The next time you feel guilty for even thinking about taking a break, remember it is only partially for your benefit. Your child will reap a great deal of the benefit as well. Small breaks and respites are guaranteed to take the edge off your tension, renew your energy, and give you a fresh dose of patience to help you pick up your care-giving duties once again. Respite is the primary mechanism you have as a family caregiver to refill your tank and thereby keep on going.

Although it may be tough to get an extended period time to work on hobbies, it may be possible to grab a few minutes here and there. It may be a small escape at best, but it is time when you can focus on something you enjoy and clear your mind. The trick is to set up a space in your home where you can retreat to for a few minutes and work on a project. Here are some ideas:

- **Music**. If playing an instrument is your hobby, don't keep it tucked away. Keep the instrument out where you can pick it up for five or ten minutes at a time. It may be the only practice you get, but with a few minutes here and there you can keep your skill up and achieve some relaxation. If listening to music is your enjoyment, an iPod is ideal because it is so portable. You can listen to it while doing chores. You can download iTunes to your computer and listen to them while you work on the computer. Music can be very soothing. Plus, many informational pod casts are available for download.

- **Art**. Art is a great escape whether you look at it or create it. If looking is your interest, keep an art book in your space so that you can look at it when you have a few minutes. If you prefer to create art, set up an easel so you can paint when you have the chance. Or use a sketch pad, and sketch using pencil or create pictures using charcoal, pen, ink, or colored pencils.

- **Writing**. I have heard about people who have written novels by getting up early and writing for one hour a day. Keep a note pad handy or carry one with you when you go out. You might get an idea when you least expect it.

- **Journaling**. Journaling is not only a great escape, but a great way to track where you are day-to-day. Journaling can also help you to get in touch with yourself. Enter one thing you are grateful for daily. *A Guided Journal for Caregivers* by Marion Karpinski, R.N., is available through amazon.com. It provides a variety of tools to help caregivers reduce stress, increase well-being, and enjoy creative expressions. It states that writing about life challenges and how we feel about them improves mental and physical health. The journal also contains a variety of exercises to help caregivers connect and express their deeper feelings through writing.

- **Surfing the web**. Google information about which you have been curious. Wikipedia is another good source of information.

- **Needlework**: The thing about needlework is that it takes up little space and is quite portable. It's easy to pick up and start and easy to get to an end point.

- **Word games and puzzles**. You can get books of word games, sudoku, and brain teasers. They are great ways to stretch your mind and change your focus.

- **Cooking**. Cooking is both creative and practical. The wonderful thing about cooking is that it is something that can be completed in a relatively short period of time. You can create something, and then you and your family can enjoy eating it.

- **Reading**. Keep a book or magazine handy both at home and in your car so that when you have a minute, or are waiting at a railroad crossing, you can do some reading.

HEALTH

Maintaining your health is very important. Some suggestions include:

- **Eat well.** Good nutrition is very important to maintain your health and energy. Keep a supply of fresh fruits, vegetables, whole wheat bread, canned tuna, dried cranberries, walnuts, olive oil, fat-free milk, and healthy snack foods. When choosing other fare, go for low-fat or fat-free food.

- **Exercise**. Exercise is one of the best stress relievers there is. Walking or running is easy to do because you can do it anywhere, anytime. An excellent aid to maintaining an exercise program is to find a partner to do it with you.

- **Monitor your health**. Have an annual checkup to keep on top of your health. Prepare for your appointment by jotting down any questions for your doctor before you go. See your dentist twice a year.

- **Vitamins**. Take a multiple vitamin and any other vitamins you may not be getting in your diet. If you are female, make sure you are getting enough calcium.

- **Wash your hands**. Hands spread germs. You pick them up from surfaces and if you then touch your eyes, nose, or mouth, you could become ill. Hand washing is one of the best ways to protect yourself during the cold and flu season. If you cough or sneeze, remember to do it in the crook of your arm.

- **Bubble bath**. A bubble bath is very soothing and relaxing. Add Epsom salts to aid in the relaxation of tired, sore muscles.

- **Yoga**. Set up a place where you can practice. Breathing with the poses is very important. If you are not familiar with yoga, sign up for a class at the YMCA, through community education, or a local community college. Recently I studied Isha Yoga, or as Sadhguru put it "Inner Engineering." I have been studying Kundalini Yoga for almost a year. Isha practices the ancient yogic principle that the body is the temple of the spirit and health is fundamental to personal and spiritual development. He emphasizes that happiness is only found within. This program is communicated on the experiential level. It opens the heart and consciousness to new dimensions of feeling, thinking, and living. Joy and inner peace can virtually eliminate stress. I learned that all that is real is this moment. We learn from the past and plan for the future, but live in this moment. No matter what happens, we can then think clearly about what is needed in the next moment. This sense of well-being can only enhance life.

- **Meditation**. Sit in a quiet place where you will not be interrupted. Make sure your back is straight. You can sit on the floor (on a pillow if you like) or in a chair with your feet flat on the floor. Breathe deeply and relax. Imagine there are three burdens on your shoulders. Visualize knocking them off as you take a deep breath. At first many, many thoughts will come to you; you'll probably feel that you are not getting anywhere and you are not feeling calm and serene. Just let the thoughts go. After awhile, you will become an observer watching yourself. When I achieved this state, I could see the bigger picture; I saw myself as a small dot, but still integrally involved with what was going on.

MINI-ESCAPES

If it's not practical to take a weekend vacation, you can get away at least for an afternoon:

- **Museums**. Visit a local museum or art gallery.

- **Overnight outings**. I have a friend who moved to a new city about 200 miles away. While our schedules don't allow us to get together for a weekend, occasionally we meet in the middle on a Friday night after work. It is less than a two-hour drive for each of us to get to the hotel. We get a room with a balcony overlooking the pool. We relax on the balcony while catching up, do our nails, and go to the dining room for dinner. After dinner, we watch an in-room movie. The next morning we enjoy breakfast together, get on the road and arrive home early afternoon. It is just one night away, but it is so refreshing that it feels like a weekend.

- **Massage**. A massage is a great way to relax and help your tired muscles at the same time.

- **Enroll in a class**. Is there something you have wanted to learn but just haven't gotten around to it? Chances are there might be a class of interest offered in a local community college or through an adult education program. Taking a class makes you commit to the project. It's another good way to escape and immerse yourself in a new experience.

PART THREE:
RESOURCES

There are several resources that are helpful in dealing with a child with a traumatic brain injury.

Web sites with information on Traumatic Brain Injury (TBI)

There are thousands of Web sites concerning brain injury. I have reviewed many of these, and have listed a small number of a variety sites which contain the most useful information. All have links to other sites, and so through this limited listing, you have access to thousands of resources.

- Brain Injury Association of America at www.biausa.org. The Brain Injury Association of America (BIAA) is the leading national organization serving and representing individuals, families, and professionals who are touched by a life-altering, often devastating, traumatic brain injury (TBI). Together with its network of more than forty chartered state affiliates, as well as hundreds of local chapters and support groups across the country, the BIAA provides information, education, and support to assist the 5.3 million Americans currently living with traumatic brain injury and their families. The state sites contain useful information about available resources within each state. The sites listed below are some of the most informational and useful:

- Washington's BIAA site is useful and has a lot of helpful informational and educational articles along with a tool kit. http://www.biawa.org/index.html

- New Jersey's BIAA site has on-line courses for educators dealing with brain injury. http://www.bianj.org/returntoschool.html

- New Mexico has a site that is very well-designed. They have a highly informative guide for understanding brain injury. http://www.braininjurynm.com

- Iowa now has a plan for coping with the different stages of brain injury. This is the first state to have a needs-assessment of brain injury. http://www.biausa.org/Iowa/

- The International Brain Injury Association at http://www.international-brain.org. The IBIA is dedicated to the development and support of multidisciplinary medical and clinical professionals, advocates, policy makers, consumers and others who work to improve outcomes and opportunities for persons with brain injury. Founded in 1993, the IBIA was created in response to the growing demand from professionals and advocates throughout the world for collaboration and more information on all aspects of brain injury, from prevention to long-term care issues.

- North American Brain Injury Society (NABIS) at http://www.nabis.org. NABIS is a society comprised of professional members involved in the care or issues surrounding brain injury. The principle mission of the organization is moving brain injury science into practice. Whether it is in the area of clinical care, research, policy, or litigation, the organization stands behind the premise that advances in science and practices based on application of the scientific evidence will ultimately provide the best outcomes for those with brain injuries and the community as a whole. Although this is a site for professionals, there are links to books and resources that may be useful.

- National Rehabilitation Information Center (NARIC) at http://www.naric.com. The NARIC Web site is a gateway to an abundance of disability and rehabilitation-oriented information organized in a variety of formats designed to make it easy to find and use. For the past twenty-five years NARIC staff members have been dedicated to providing direct, personal, and high-quality information services to anyone throughout the country. As you search through this site, you're actually going through more than twenty years of collecting, organizing, and maintaining the most current information in the field. What started as a small collection now includes more than 70,000 documents and journal articles.

- The National Institute on Disability and Rehabilitation Research (NIDRR) at http://www.ed.gov/about/offices/list/osers/nidrr/index.html. NIDRR provides leadership and support for a comprehensive program of research related to the rehabilitation of individuals with disabilities. All of our programmatic efforts are aimed at improving the lives of individuals with disabilities from birth through adulthood.

- National Resources Center for Traumatic Brain Injury at http://www.neuro.pmr.vcu,edu. This site provides relevant, practical information for professionals, persons with brain injury, and family members. Guides and books are available. It's part of the Virginia Commonwealth University, VCU Health System.

- National Dissemination Center for Children with Disabilities (NICHCY) at http://nichcy.org. NICHCY contains a wealth of information on disabilities in infants, toddlers, children, and youth. This includes IDEA, which is the law authorizing special education, No Child Left Behind (as it relates to children with disabilities), and research-based information on effective educational practices.

- National Institute of Neurologic Disorders and Stroke (NINDS) at http://www.nlm.nih.gov/medlineplus/medlineplus.html. The mission of NINDS is to reduce the burden of neurological disease—a burden borne by every age group, by every segment of society, by people all over the world. Although this site may be clinical in nature, there is information that may be helpful to families. Use the search function to find brain injury.

- Brain Injury Resource Center at http://www.headinjury.com. This site contains basic information about head injury. It has a tool kit listing a multitude of resources.

- Virtual Hospital—A Guide for Family and Friends at http://vh.org. This site is part of the University of Iowa and is concise, easy to navigate, and has all the basics.

- SURVIVAL GUIDE ON-LINE BOOK by Dr. Glen Johnson, Clinical Neuropsychologist at http://www.tbiguide.com. Dr. Johnson published this information because he said nearly all of the survivors of a traumatic head injury and their families with whom he has worked have had one complaint: There is nothing written that explains head injury in clear, easy to understand language. Most say the available material is too medical or too difficult to read. The goal of this online book is to better prepare the head injured person and family for the long road ahead.

- Defense and Veterans Brain Injury Center (DVBIC) at http://dvbic.org. DVBIC serves active duty military, their dependents and veterans with traumatic brain injury (TBI) through state-of-the-art medical care, innovative clinical research initiatives and educational programs.

- The New Mexico Traumatic Brain Injury Resource Manual Project at http://www.nmaging.state.nm.us/HTML/index.html. This Web site is the online version of the New Mexico Brain Injury Resources Manual. It is organized so the section topics may be extracted, printed, distributed, and used as needed by individuals, their families, case managers, discharge planners, and other professionals. It is a comprehensive guide of information and the Web site map may be the easiest tool to use to navigate the site. A print version of the Web site is available in English, Spanish, and in an audio Navajo version on CD.

- Family Care Network at http://www.rehabmedicine.pitt.edu. The Family Care Network provides access to important information and resources for people with traumatic brain injury and their families. The site is designed to deliver pertinent information at each stage of recovery. It starts with defining TBI, and then leads you through rehabilitation, the initial stages of returning home and re-entering the community, living with TBI and, finally, legal considerations. A part of the University of Pittsburgh, the site contains lot of unique, practical information and tips.

- TBI Help Desk for Caregivers at http://www.tbihelp.org. This site contains a lot of useful articles and information, and is easy to navigate. It is owned and operated by Jamaica Hospital Medical Center and sponsored by United Hospital Fund.

FACILITIES

Facilities around the country are listed on the head injury Web site at http://www.headinjury.com/rehabfacility.htm.

Substance Abuse Organizations

It became apparent in talking with health professionals that both families and higher functioning injured people turn to substance abuse to "deal with" and/or "escape" their problems, stresses, etc. There are several substance abuse organizations that may be helpful:

- Drug and Alcohol Resource Center; Nationwide Alcohol and Drug Addiction Rehab Information. They provide help for the Family with alcohol, drug addiction, and substance abuse. While this Web site is provided by a treatment facility in Florida, they do have a lot of helpful and useful information. For immediate information, call 1–800–784–6776 or visit http://www.addict-help.com.

- Alcoholics Anonymous. Alcoholics Anonymous is a voluntary, worldwide fellowship of men and women from all walks of life who meet together to attain and maintain sobriety. The only requirement for membership is a desire to stop drinking. There are no dues or fees for A.A. membership. A.A. does not allow people with other addictions to join, only alcoholics. Their Web site has useful information. You can find an A.A. office in your area on their Web site or look for Alcoholics Anonymous in any telephone directory. In most urban areas, a central A.A. office, or intergroup, staffed mainly by volunteer A.A.s, will be happy to answer your questions and/or put you in touch with those who can. Visit http://www.alcohol-ics-anonymous.org.

• National Institute on Alcohol Abuse and Alcoholism. This is a subsection of the National Institutes of Health. It contains information that has more of a clinical/medical bend but may provide useful information to the general public. Visit http://alcoholism.about.com.

• ABOUT: Alcoholism and Substance Abuse. The ABOUT Web site is associated with the New York Times Company and serves as a clearing house for information. Go to the site and insert "alcoholism" and "substance abuse" into the search option. It will give you many links to various aspects of the subject you indicated. Visit http://www.about.com.

• MedlinePlus. MedlinePlus directs you to information to help answer health questions. MedlinePlus brings together authoritative information from the National Library of Medicine (NLM), the National Institutes of Health (NIH), and other government agencies and health-related organizations. Pre-formulated MEDLINE searches are included in MedlinePlus and give easy access to medical journal articles. MedlinePlus also has extensive information about drugs, an illustrated medical encyclopedia, interactive patient tutorials, and latest health news.

ESTATE PLANNING:
INFORMATION ON WILLS
AND SPECIFIC NEEDS
TRUSTS

Note: The National Information Center for Children and Youth with Disabilities (www. nichcy.org) in Washington D.C. has some very comprehensive information on estate planning for parents of a child with a disability. I have summarized the information listed there, and it was reviewed for accuracy by a lawyer and accountant. However, laws vary from state to state and change over time, so the information provided should be used only for informational purposes. I strongly recommend you consult a lawyer for assistance.

One of the most pressing and nagging questions that worries parents with a son or daughter with a brain injury is, "What will happen to my child when I am no longer able to provide care?" It turns out that this can be a complex question with complicated answers. The individual situation and family resources determine the best plan of action. That is why it is so important to have an attorney who is familiar with estate planning for parents who have a child with a disability. In my own situation, T's sister agreed to assume care for T when I can no longer care for her. I have established trusts to assure that T will have the financial resources to live out her life in a comfortable way. But this is something that requires study, research, and consultation with an attorney to determine what is best for each situation. Make sure your trust includes an alternate caregiver in case something happens to the one you have chosen.

One of the first big questions to be answered is concerning public assistance support for your dependent, and whether or not your son or daughter receives (or may one day need to depend on) government benefits such as Supplemental Security Insurance (SSI), subsidized housing, personal attendant care, or Medicaid. If your child does receive (or may one day need to depend on) government benefits, then it is most important to create a special estate plan that does not negate his or her eligibility for those benefits.

While the services available through government benefit programs may be substantial, the actual cash benefits are generally quite small and force the individual to live way below the poverty level. In 2007, the maximum Federal SSI monthly payment for a child with a disability in Michigan was $623. This means that, for an individual with a disability to have any type of meaningful lifestyle, the family or local charities have to provide supplemental assistance.

If a person with a disability is relying on governmental benefit programs as a mainstay of support, inheriting even a small amount of money could disqualify her from being eligible to receive those benefits. Let's look at the example of Lisa, a woman with a brain injury who is unable to work or be responsible for herself in day-to-day activities. Her parents passed away and she inherited $50,000. But that means she is no longer eligible for governmental benefit programs and must now provide for her own medical care, which includes the considerable cost of medicine, personal care attendants, physical therapy, and doctor visits. She is living in a group home which will begin to charge her for residency and the services she receives there. This will continue until all but $2,000 (SSI resource limit) of the inheritance is gone. At this point, she again becomes eligible for government benefits and is re-instated after a waiting period during which she uses up the last of her inheritance. Now there are no funds left to pay for whatever supplemental needs she might have: education, over-the-counter medicines, dental care beyond what is covered by government benefits, trips to see her sister or other family-members. Government benefits do not cover these types of expenses, and Lisa's parents are no longer here to do so. The irony of the situation is that, while an inheritance should ordinarily improve a person's lifestyle, this one has worsened Lisa's in the end. Let's start at the beginning and review the things that, as a parent of a child with a brain injury, you should keep in mind when doing estate planning.

CREATING A WILL

A will ensures that the assets of a deceased parent are distributed according to his or her wishes. Without a will, the parent's assets would be distributed according to the law of the state, called the law of interstacy. Although interstacy laws vary from state to state, in general they provide that some percent of the decedent's assets pass to the surviving spouse and the remainder are divided equally among the children. Writing a will is very important because the laws of interstacy are rarely the most desirable way to pass property on to one's heirs. More importantly, have this will written by a lawyer familiar with disabilities because when a child with a disability is involved, there are special planning concerns. It's important to remember when preparing a will that not all your assets are governed by a will. For example, joint property with right of survivorship passes independently of a will. Also, life insurance is paid directly to the person named beneficiary. This is also true for employee pension plans.

Another very important thing to know is that a will does not protect your assets from being probated. A will is essentially your statement to a probate judge on how you want the judge to see that the probate assets are distributed. A will in probate can result in assets being tied up, the need for legal assistance and, hence, more expense. Personal property such as jewelry, clothing, furniture, and household items should be distributed independently of other more valuable assets such as stocks, bonds, and property. A will only goes into effect upon the person's death and can be modified at any time before then.

When you begin planning, you should have a good idea of what your dependent with a disability will require after you are no longer able to care for him or her. A professional assessment as to future requirements might be warranted to determine how much needs may change in future years. Remember you can change your estate plan for your dependent as more information about the future becomes available.

You will then need to consider your financial affairs, your son or daughter's living arrangements and potential earning power, as well as governmental benefits he or she may need and are eligible to receive. Be very careful to consider all the options so as to not put your child in a situation where an inheritance will do more harm than good in the long run. The NICHCY Web site information suggests four approaches to establishing a will:

- Disinherit your son or daughter with a disability because this could be the best thing for them in order to maintain state and federal supports after your death.

- Leave your son or daughter with a disability an outright gift if he or she is not receiving or expecting to receive government benefits and if he or she can handle the financial responsibilities. If you want to leave a gift to support your dependent, a trust may be the preferred route.

- Leave a morally obliged gift to another of your children with no disability. Suppose you tell your daughter Sue that you are leaving all the financial assets to her, but that you expect her to use half of the assets in the way she sees best for Lisa's care so as not to disqualify Lisa from her governmental benefits, but this has some risks involved. This is a moral obligation and, legally, the assets belong to Sue to spend as she wishes. But even if Sue did wish to carry out your wishes, she may come upon circumstances making it impossible to fulfill those wishes. For example if Sue or one of her children becomes ill and in great financial need, Sue may feel pressure to use the money for her own family. Also if Sue dies before Lisa, Sue's family may not be willing to carry out the parent's wishes. Finally if Sue and her husband divorce, some of the money may be lost in a divorce settlement.

- Establish a discretionary or special needs trust for your son or daughter with a disability which often is the most effective way to help them. The trust will not disqualify them from the governmental benefits for which they might otherwise be eligible.

Special Needs Trust

The only reliable method to make sure an inheritance reaches a person with a disability is through a Special Needs Trust (SNT). The SNT is developed to manage resources while maintaining the individual's eligibility for public assistance benefits. The family leaves resources to the trust which is managed by a trustee who has the absolute discretion to provide whatever assistance is required on behalf of the person with the disability. While government agencies recognize special needs trusts, they have imposed some very stringent rules and regulations upon them. So if you are contemplating an SNT, it is very important to have an attorney who is knowledgeable about SNTs and current government benefit programs. One wrong word or phrase can make the difference between an inheritance that really benefits the person with a disability and one that causes the person to lose access to a wide range of needed services and assistance. The trustee should never give the person with the disability more income or resources than permitted by the government and make sure the resources are used for supplementary purposes only; it should add to the things provided by the government benefit program, not supplant (replace) them. This would be for items other than the person's food, clothing, and shelter such as medical care, telephone bills, education, and entertainment. The trust also provides instructions for the person's final arrangement and determines who should receive the remainder (what is left over) of the trust after the individual with the disability dies. The trust also provides choices for successor trustees: people or organizations that might be able to take a personal interest in the welfare of the person with the disability and protects the trust against creditors or government agencies trying to obtain funds to pay for debts of the person or the family.

Testamentary or Intervivos Trust

Attorneys used to advise parents of an individual with a disability to prepare their Last Wills and Testaments and include a Testamentary Special Needs Trust. Upon the death of the parents, the wills would be probated, and the special needs trust would be created. Today, most attorneys who are experienced in estate planning for persons with disabilities will advise the family to prepare an Intervivos Special Needs Trust. Intervivos simply means that the trust functions now, while the parents are still living. As a "living" trust, it should not be confused with the modern estate planning tool for the family's main estate, the Family Revocable Living Trust. These are two very separate trusts. The Family Living Trust is designed to avoid probate, reduce estate taxes, and make for a smoother estate distribution. The Intervivos Special Needs Trust's sole function is to look after the future of the person with the disability.

Revocable or Irrevocable

Next, you have to decide whether to make the trust final with no future changes or to be able to make some changes. With a Revocable trust, the major consequence is that the government considers the trust to be part of the parent's estate. Therefore, when the parents die, everything in the special needs trust is included in their estate for tax purposes and for potential lawsuits. What happens if someone sues your estate after you are gone? The assets in your special needs trust could be lost in such a lawsuit. If you make your trust Irrevocable, it means that any assets you place in it will remain there for the benefit of the person with the disability. It is separate from your estate with its own tax number. Any assets that you place in the trust cannot be touched by your creditors for debts, taxes, and so on. Neither can the trust be touched by any creditors of the person with the disability. Of course if you make your trust irrevocable, you cannot change it at a later date.

There are many things to consider and many questions to answer that do not have quick, easy answers. Do a Google search using the phrase "Providing a meaningful life for a child with a disability after your death" to find books, links, and other information. Again, an attorney knowledgeable about estate planning for parents with a child with a disability is a must. Also, it is very important that the parents discuss their ideas between themselves and have a general idea of what their goals are before consulting an attorney. With planning and legal assistance, you can feel relieved that your child with a disability will live comfortably without you.

EPILOGUE

▼

January 19, 2008

On December 28, 2007, I took Tania to Beaumont Hospital's emergency room. She had fallen at home and complained of lower back pain. They ended up admitting her. The fall was due to an increased lack of balance. There is a slight indentation in the tailbone. She could not open her eyes and was having great trouble swallowing.

Tania is now being transferred to a rehabilitation facility called Rainbow. Apparently, fifteen years plus following brain trauma, scar tissue sometimes develops in the brain and some gains can become lost. Slightly before her admission to Beaumont, I had hired a medical case manager because Tania's care was becoming overwhelming. Our medical case manager contacted Rainbow for us. This is a new rehabilitation hospital in Farmington Hills, fairly close to our home. It is Rainbow's goal to bring these gains back or help her adapt to her new situation.

Tania's sense of balance is no better than when she went into Beaumont two weeks ago, and it is currently not safe for her to return home. I am not particularly hopeful she will walk again, as her balance is still really skewed. She still cannot open her eyes. The great medical minds say they can do nothing more for her.

Tania's spirit of braveness and courage is faltering. She is very sad because she had her hopes up on coming home. I am tired and frustrated because I am afraid her depression could deepen. All she wants is to be home where she left her heart but we are not equipped to deal with her now. She is not safe because of the falling. I see her try to smile and remember her laughter and feel a cloud of doom descending. I hear one of her songs and the actual ache in my chest is stronger. What will become of her? Will she ever have a place in this world? Will I ever have a place without her?

Both Tania and myself as women are embarking on a new journey which is only now becoming delineated. Our journey reflects my early dream of loving Tania, accepting her, and letting her be. I am discovering who I am besides Tania's mother. I think this is important for each mother: self-discovery, other than the role of Mom. I am also allowing Tania to discover who she is in her world. I know I have pushed her too hard to be like "us", which is not acceptance.

Despite the fact that she struggles with a traumatic brain injury, Tania has made the most of her life, and I will be forever grateful that I have been blessed with such a beautiful daughter.

Mary Burgess-Smith

Bibliography

Barry, P., & Riley, J. 1987. Adult norms for the Kaufman hand movements test and a single-subject design for acute brain injured rehabilitation. *Journal of Clinical and Experimental Neuropsychology, 449.*

Davidson, Jeff, MBA, CMC, *The Complete Idiot's Guide to Managing Stress.* United States: Alpha Books, 1999

Karpman, T., Wolfe, J., & Vargo J. 1986. The psychological adjustment of adult clients and their parents following closed head injury. *Journal of Applied Rehabilitation Counseling, 17, 28–33.*

Lezak, M. 1986. Psychological implications of traumatic brain damage for the patient's family. *Rehabilitation Psychology, 31, 242–247.*

Mitiguy, J.S., Thompson, G.T., & Wasco, J. 1990. *Understanding Brain Injury.* Massachusetts: New Medico Head Injury System.

Reese, R. 1983. How some families cope and why some families do not. *Journal of Head Trauma Rehabilitation. 3. 72–77.*

Ridley, B. 1990. Family response in head injury: Denial of hope for a future? *Social Science and Medicine, 4, 555–561.*

Schoen, Barb. 2007. Families and Disability: 1–14.

Spanbock, P. 1987. Understanding head injury from the families' perspective. *Cognitive Rehabilitation, 5: 12–14.*

Spordone, R., Kral, M., Gerald, M., & Katz. 1984. Evidence of a "command performance syndrome" in the significant others of the victims of severe traumatic brain injury. *International Journal of Neuropsychology, 6: 183–185.*

Sternberg, Esther, M. *The Balance Within: The Science Connecting Health and Emotions.* New York, New York: W.H. Freeman and Company, 2001.

Tarter, S. 1990. Factors affecting adjustment of parents of head trauma victims. *Archives of Clinical Neuropsychology, 5, 15–22.*

Zarski, J., DePompei, R., & Zack, A. 1988. Traumatic Head Injury: Dimensions of family responsibility. *Journal of Head Trauma Rehabilitation, 4, 31–41.*

978-0-595-48718-9
0-595-48718-1

www.ingramcontent.com/pod-product-compliance
Lightning Source LLC
Chambersburg PA
CBHW030753180526
45163CB00003B/1007